Fever Hospital

Fever Hospital

A History of
Fairfield Infectious
Diseases Hospital

W. K. Anderson

MELBOURNE UNIVERSITY PRESS

MELBOURNE UNIVERSITY PRESS
PO Box 278, Carlton South, Victoria 3053, Australia
info@mup.unimelb.edu.au
www.mup.com.au

First published 2002

Designed by Lauren Statham, Alice Graphics
Typeset in 11 point Bembo by Syarikat Seng Teik Sdn. Bhd., Malaysia
Printed in Australia by Brown Prior Anderson

National Library of Australia Cataloguing-in-Publication entry

Anderson, William Keys, 1953– .
   Fever hospital: a history of Fairfield Infectious Diseases Hospital.
   Bibliography.
   Includes index.
   ISBN 0 522 84964 4.

   1. Fairfield Hospital (Melbourne, Vic.)—History. 2. Communicable
   diseases—Hospitals—Victoria—Melbourne—History. I. Title.

362.11099451

Publication was assisted by generous contributions from the
Alfred Hospital, Melbourne and the Victorian Infectious Diseases
Research Laboratory.

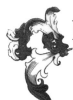

Foreword

T HE HISTORY OF Fairfield Hospital might seem at first glance to be that of a small institution which dealt with disappearing diseases. Precisely the opposite is the case. Infectious diseases have evolved and multiplied. Pathogenic microbes are masters of the phenomenon called 'change' that is so often lauded in other contexts. Fairfield Hospital thrived on the changing challenges of infections, as has the discipline of infectious diseases.

In the words of Dr William Anderson, the author of this book, the hospital has a 'rich and multifaceted history'. Although mooted as far back as 1869, it was not until 1904 that the hospital was opened to patients. The cavalcade of infections that passed through its portals began with scarlet fever and diphtheria and steadily increased over the decades. For a large part of its existence Fairfield Hospital treated all types of infections, whether contagious or otherwise. Expertise in research and public health developed early, gaining national and international recognition, including the creation of the Macfarlane Burnet Centre for Medical Research (now the Macfarlane Burnet Institute). Locally, the hospital was the principle centre for infectious diseases. Undergraduate student teaching in the discipline of infectious dis-eases began in the 1950s. Postgraduate training began soon after the formation of the Australasian Society for Infectious Diseases in 1976. Dr John Forbes, the Medical Superintendent at that time, was the co-founder and inaugural president of the society.

The hospital repeatedly rose to the demands of new infections, the most recent of which was HIV/AIDS, its last major challenge. The longstanding ethos and experience of managing patients with infections was called upon in abundance to deal with this new world-wide epidemic. The subsequent dedication and honing of skills led to what became widely known as the 'Fairfield culture of care', an approach involving medical, nursing, allied health and pastoral care. The combination of this with high levels of active research led to international renown in the field.

Effective treatment for those living with HIV/AIDS had just begun to make a real impact when the government of the day announced the closure of Fairfield Hospital. This was a less than pleasant undertaking for both patients and staff. The trauma induced by the announcement was compounded by the haste with which the government intended to shut down the hospital. In the event, they were thwarted to some extent by underestimation of the medical complexity and the stalwart character of both patients and staff. Close it they did, but the legacy of a proud institution lives on.

The dispersal of the patients, staff, students, clinical services and laboratories was predictably chaotic. The physical components have been gradually re-established in Melbourne's university teaching hospitals. It remains unclear as to whether the present access, adequacy and level of care are equivalent. As in the case of the French Revolution, we are still waiting to see if it has all been worthwhile. However, in the aftermath of death there is always a legacy. In this case there are many positive aspects, ranging from ground-breaking findings of research through grateful patients to a small army of doctors, nurses and allied health personnel whose culture of care and infectious diseases training will benefit the community for years to come.

My own involvement in this long-awaited book began in 1987 when I called together those with an interest in the hospital's history, and unwittingly became the founder of the Fairfield Hospital Historical Collection Committee. The endeavours of these loyal and hard-working members led to what has become one of the best curated and most comprehensive and admired hospital museum collections. The archives and artefacts have been a major source in the writing of this excellent history. However, the most important step came shortly before the close of the hospital when Bill Anderson agreed to write its history Bill has the ideal background, from the viewpoint of a biased Fairfield person. He has an understanding of hospitals, having worked in one, and he is an experienced and highly regarded historian. His book tells us a lot more than what happened and when; it gives an insight into what it was like for all those involved in the Fairfield experience.

Dr Bryan Speed
Infectious Diseases Physician, Fairfield Hospital, 1974–1996
(now at Austin and Repatriation Medical Centre)

To all the patients and staff of Fairfield Hospital from its foundation to its closure, and to everyone who through the years has supported Fairfield's work of caring, healing and research.

Contents

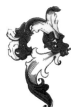

Illustrations

Unless otherwise stated, photographs are from the Fairfield Hospital Archives, Austin Hospital, Melbourne.

Acknowledgements

In researching and writing this history of Fairfield Hospital I have received generous and enthusiastic support from a great many people who have been associated in some way with the Hospital over the years, and I would like to gratefully acknowledge this assistance.

In particular I would like to thank Jillian McCloy, Gwen McPherson, Barbara Rossall-Wynne, Dr A. Murray Sandland, Dr Bryan Speed and Dr Di Tibbits who, as members of the Reference Group established by the Hospital to support this work, provided unstinting support, guidance and encouragement.

I am deeply indebted to the Fairfield Hospital Historical Collection Committee (Margaret Elliott-Commons, Dr Robert Grogan, Lois Jefcotte, Gwen McPherson, William (Bill) Phillips, Chris Richards, Barbara Rossall-Wynne, Dr A. Murray Sandland, Valerie Seager, Pena Soccio and Dr B Speed) and to the numerous staff, patients and supporters who helped in many ways with oral histories, photographs, media clippings, old nurses uniforms and certificates. The Fairfield Hospital Archive and Museum, located at the Austin Hospital, is a remarkable and historically important collection. It is a tribute to the immense dedication and hard work of its voluntary supporters over many years; I note in particular the contributions of curators Barbara Rossall-Wynne and Maja Bercloux.

Other medical and scientific staff who assisted include Dr B. Dwyer, Professor I. Gust, Dr A. Kucers, Dr R. Lucas, Joseph Manitta, Dr A. Mijch, Dr H. Newton-John, Robert Pringle and Dr A. Yung. Members of the nursing staff have displayed a particular enthusiasm for this project and I would like to acknowledge the contributions of the Fairfield Past Nurses Association and of Val Seager, Vera Westley, the late Vivian Bullwinkle and the late Gwen Burbidge.

Others who provided various forms of important assistance include Dr Chris Brook, Graeme Houghton, Mrs K. Kerin (Nursing Home Supervisor), Dave O'Brien, Chris Richards, Jennifer Rusciano (Librarian), Dr Michael Stanford and Jan Watson.

Finally I would like to acknowledge the assistance, support and encouragement of my wife, Esther Anderson, who by fortunate coincidence is a medical writer by profession.

Introduction

I should welcome the sick to my feast,
For they are God's joy.
Let the poor sit with Jesus at the highest place,
And the sick dance with the angels.
St Brigid's Grace[1]

Over the proud new city of Melbourne hung a miasmic curse of neglected sanitation and human suffering, especially among young children who died in agony and in great numbers. The scandal was preventable: several English towns had already installed efficient water and sewerage works. But Melbourne, wealthy Melbourne, simply would not face up to the problem. It almost seemed that its citizens preferred to live among filth and watch unconcernedly as their weaker brethren were carried off by so-called 'zymotic' diseases . . . Gold-rush Melbourne had no infectious diseases hospital or children's hospital. Victims of disease were mostly treated at home by visiting doctors, or left to die . . .
Michael Cannon, *Melbourne After the Gold Rush*[2]

From time immemorial, infectious disease has been one of humankind's greatest fears. Even before we had any real understanding of how infections spread, the sick were feared and a primitive concept of contagion exerted a strong influence. Long before we had any comprehension of the infection process, the sick were pitied and shunned as much as, if not more than, they were cared for. Infectious diseases have always terrified—and at times have nearly destroyed—our species. Allusions to specific epidemics and pandemics permeate our literature and indeed our whole culture. One of the first rhymes learnt by generations of Anglo-Celtic children comes down to us from the aptly named Black Death of the fourteenth century:

Ring-a-ring o' roses,
A pocket full of posies,
A-tishoo! A-tishoo!
We all fall down.[3]

1

And fall down we did in huge numbers, to a wide variety of infectious diseases—often suffering such great agonies that death was indeed a welcome relief.

The 'primitive' fears which infectious diseases inspired in our ancestors are by no means vanquished in our modern, sophisticated, scientific world. In recent years the fear of coming into contact with people who are HIV positive has at times become almost hysterical—who can forget the film of young children being stopped from entering primary schools by 'concerned' parents? Even some hospitals allowed emotion and ancient fears to so cloud their collective reasons and sense of mission that they refused to treat HIV patients.

Given the grave importance with which we have invested infectious diseases down through the ages, it is hardly surprising that the Holy Book of Christianity and Judaism contains one of the earliest descriptions of infectious

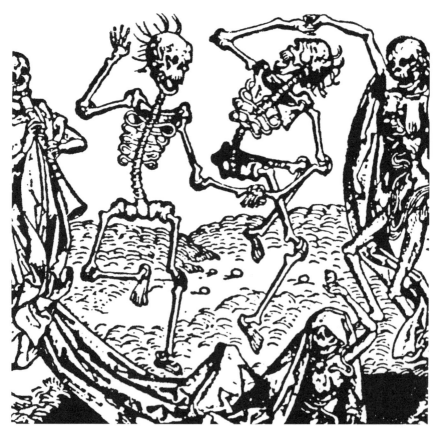

A macabre contemporary depiction of the dance of the Black Death through fourteenth-century Europe.

disease (leprosy—Hansen's disease) and provides not only detailed advice on recognition, care and treatment of disease but also a series of rules regarding quarantine controls. Leviticus chapter 13 says:

1 And the Lord spake unto Moses and Aaron, saying,

2 When a man shall have in the skin of his flesh a rising, a scab, or bright spot, and it be in the skin of his flesh *like* the plague of leprosy; then he shall be brought unto Aaron the priest, or unto one of his sons the priests:

3 And the priest shall look on the plague in the skin of the flesh: and *when* the hair the plague is turned white, and the plague in sight *be* deeper than the skin of his flesh, it *is a* plague of leprosy; and the priest shall look on him, and pronounce him unclean . . .

45 And the leper in whom the plague *is*, his clothes shall be rent, and his head bare, and he shall put a covering upon his upper lip, and shall cry, Unclean, unclean.

46 And all the days wherein the plague *shall be* in him he shall be defiled; he *is* unclean: he shall dwell alone; without the camp *shall* his habitation be . . .

50 And the priest shall look upon the plague, and shut up *it that hath* the plague seven days.

A good deal of this is sensible medical advice—although some of the detailed instructions given in later verses regarding the important role that chickens and lambs played in combating infection create a few doubts.

One recent commentator on our unwelcome but unavoidable relationship with infectious diseases has drawn attention to the complexity of the process:

The history of epidemics is the history of wars and wanderings, of famine and drought and of man's exposure to inhospitable surroundings . . . But epidemics have also occurred when man has *not* been off his guard. Poliomyelitis has been a killing disease where standards of hygiene are highest, and many diseases, such as measles and the common cold, flourish in the most civilized communities. Man's attempt to manipulate his resources have often brought him infection . . . he got bovine tuberculosis from his cattle, brucellosis from his goats, and 'Q' fever from his sheep . . . he imported smallpox in bales of cotton, anthrax in cargoes of hides or bones, psittacosis in parrots and innumerable salmonellae have crossed the oceans in his ships.[4]

To die in one's bed after one's allotted life-span holds few terrors for most people, but disease often kills in such a non-discriminatory manner— or, even worse, concentrates its dreaded energies on our children—that we have often resorted to supernatural explanations for these horrendous impositions. The idea that infectious diseases are some kind of divine punishment for our 'sins' has long been unfashionable, but the moralistic comments made by some people when it became clear that HIV/AIDS was, in most parts

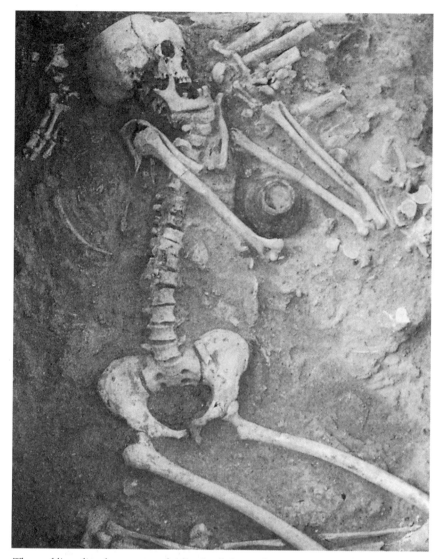

The world's earliest-known case of polio: the skeleton of a young woman excavated from a 1500 BC tomb in south-eastern Arabia.

of the world, primarily a homosexual disease—the so called 'Gay Plague'—suggest that the idea that infectious disease has its roots in the 'wrath of God' or the diabolic plots of Satan are never very far below the surface.

Like death and taxes, disease is always with us. We can all expect—as one of life's very few certainties—that we will suffer from some form of infectious disease during our lifetime. At any given moment, millions of people throughout the world are sick from an infectious disease, and even as I write this sentence someone, somewhere, has just died from an infectious disease. Some infectious diseases are rare and exotic, others are so prevalent that we have incorporated this characteristic into their vernacular name—the 'common cold', for example. Such common infectious diseases are described as being *endemic*. When the number of people suffering from any particular disease increases very markedly over a short time, we describe the disease as being an *epidemic*. An epidemic that affects a whole country or the whole world is described as a *pandemic* (from Greek—'all the people'). We often still refer to epidemics and pandemics by the ancient—and still horror-laden word—plague.

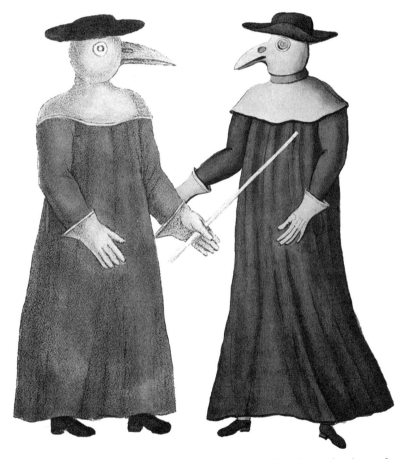

Costumes worn by doctors in the quarantined areas of Marseilles during the plague of 1720. The beak carried spices to purify the air the doctor breathed, and the wands allowed the patient's pulse to be taken without direct touching.

The treatment of infectious diseases has only in relatively recent times become both humane and rational. In Chapter 1 we examine the state of health and medical treatment in Victoria in the second part of the nineteenth century and how this led to establishing the infectious diseases hospital which is the subject—the hero—of our study, but it is worth giving a brief sketch of the development of hospital care prior to this period.

The word 'hospital' derives from the Latin *hospitium*, which means a place where guests are received. Health has always been an important concern in all human societies. We know that ancient societies worshipped gods of healing and that in Ancient Greece, some four thousand years before Christ was born, temples of deities such as Aesculapius provided facilities for treating the sick, and physicians' shops operated. In Rome, hospitals called *valetudinera* were established, and evidence from Pompeii suggests the existence of facilities similar to our modern convalescent hospital. Indeed, the Romans are generally credited with having been the originators of the modern hospital. In 355 CE, when the first Christian emperor came to power in Rome, he immediately closed all 'pagan' hospitals and encouraged the Church to take over responsibility for the building and maintenance of hospitals. Within a short time the Church was responsible for all the hospitals in Western Europe. Many monastic orders opened hospitals, and a number of religious orders were founded, specifically devoted to caring for the sick—for example, the Knights Hospitallers and the St Augustine nuns (the term 'sister' is still applied to nurses). Coe in his *Sociology of Medicine* noted:

> Work carried out among the sick was regarded as a righteous act based on the Christian ethic of charity to the sick and suffering. Volunteers who attended to the sick regarded their work as a means to their salvation rather than as an act of healing.[5]

Similar developments occurred in Muslim and other non-Christian parts of the world, and it is fair to say that the care of people's spiritual needs and their physical needs in time of sickness were, and to some extent remain even today, very closely linked.

By the seventeenth century, after more than a millennium of religious 'monopoly' of hospital construction and administration, most hospitals were becoming secularly based—although some remained and continue to be religiously based. People were beginning to recognise that hospitals were not simply responsible for custodial patient care but had three related and equally important functions—healing, research and teaching.[6] Until the late nineteenth century, hospitals were places of great danger for patients due to prevailing standards of poor cleanliness and hygiene in the community and ignorance about the dangers of cross infection. Wards were usually dirty, poorly ventilated and overcrowded, often the beds were infested with lice, and neither bedding nor patients were washed. Indeed hospitals were seen as places of last resort and mainly catered for homeless and hopeless cases. A study of early influences on the development of Australian hospitals presents a horrifying sketch of pre-modern hospital conditions:

> . . . patients were often put two in a bed, without the choice of companion . . . The wards were filled with patients suffering form a wide variety of illnesses, particularly infectious diseases. Thus, a patient with tuberculosis might find as a bedmate a person with a gangrenous limb or a woman about to give birth.[7]

When white settlers first invaded Australia in January 1788, they brought with them a host of infectious diseases that were endemic in Western Europe but previously unknown in Australia. Infectious diseases wrought havoc with these pioneering settlers, but their sufferings paled in comparison with the devastating toll that the newly introduced 'European' diseases took on the indigenous Aboriginal population, who had no acquired resistance to them. It is generally accepted that, more than any other factor, it was the introduction of infectious diseases such as measles and syphilis which demoralised and in many cases destroyed Aboriginal culture and society throughout Australia.

The first hospital in Australia opened at Dawe's Point in 1796, and 'unsanitary and overcrowded conditions causing cross infection were . . . prevalent'.[8] The standard of health care had improved little, if at all, by the time the Port Phillip settlement was established in the mid-1830s. Cannon, in his history of early Melbourne, provided a colourful and shocking account of hospital conditions in the early years of the colony:

> The first so-called hospital in Melbourne was a frail weatherboard building on the Western Market Reserve, near the watch house and police office. Originally it had been erected by merchant Francis Nodin for use as a storeroom. No separation of patients suffering from serious illnesses was possible in the cramped quarters.[9]

Dr Patrick Cussen was appointed in 1837 as the first Assistant Colonial Surgeon in Melbourne. (In 1838 he conducted, without anaesthetic, what was probably Melbourne's first surgical operation—he amputated the penis of convict William Bone, who was suffering from venereal disease.) In 1840 Dr Cussen recorded his opinion of the 'sad state' of the government hospital. Sometimes patients had to sleep on the floor, and their bedding rotted due to water lying under the floor. The building was draughty and the cold was 'frequently intolerable'.

Dysentery, syphilis and rheumatism were prevalent. Doctors could do little against most diseases, though smallpox could be prevented by vaccination. The people of Melbourne were offered smallpox vaccination early in 1840, which prevented major outbreaks. A fever, presumed to be typhoid, spread through Melbourne early in 1841, causing the death of many babies. Some government aid was made available through the town's private doctors, but this was insufficient to alleviate much of the suffering. Small wonder then that by the middle of the century community demands were growing for improvements to sanitary, medical and hospital facilities. These demands led, in time, to the establishment of Fairfield Hospital.

It is clearly impossible here to do full justice to the rich and multi-faceted history of a large and complex hospital like Fairfield. In touching upon the major events, themes and important developments, I hope that those readers who are not familiar with the hospital gain some feeling for its spirit and achievements, and that those who are—either as patients, staff or visitors—recognise the hospital they knew, and in many cases loved and respected. This book is intended to mark—and to celebrate—the work and achievements of Fairfield Hospital from its opening in 1904 to its closure in 1996. The hospital's history is also a history of the treatment of infectious diseases in Victoria in the twentieth century, and therefore a significant chapter in the history of our state and indeed our nation. It is an important and in many ways a magnificent story.

Fever Hospital
1890–1918

Diseases desperate grown,
By desperate appliances are relieved
Or not at all.

Hamlet IV, iii.

B EFORE DESCRIBING THE emergence and early development of Queen's Memorial Hospital, later Fairfield Hospital, it is necessary to sketch a brief history of infectious disease in Australia and in particular in Melbourne. It would be difficult to overstate the horrendous effects of infectious disease during the pioneer era; the toll on human life and happiness claimed by infectious diseases constituted a dark cloud hanging over the whole community. The fact that infectious diseases exerted a particularly heavy toll on the most vulnerable members of the community—the young and the indigenous people (who had little or no resistance to diseases introduced by white settlers)—makes their depredations particularly tragic and poignant. The recognition, understanding of causes and treatment of infectious diseases has been a very gradual one, although the twentieth century saw an astonishing rate of progress.

There can be little doubt that the Australians who have suffered most from the results of infectious diseases are the Indigenous Australians. Indeed their lack of resistance and susceptibility to introduced diseases resulted in the extinction of many of the Aboriginal tribes and at times appeared to threaten the very existence of the Aboriginal peoples. This devastation was rendered even worse when the discovery of gold in the early 1850s led to a further flood of European and Asian settlers who introduced yet more infectious diseases which played havoc with both Aboriginal and colonist Australians.

It has been noted that 'disease patterns in Australia are closely linked with the country's history, the two areas of study combining to provide a fascinating story of introduced disease, past, present and future'[1] and there is no doubt that this is true. One historian of infectious diseases in Australia has described this process well:

> When considering the introduction of disease into Australia, we can see a trend linked to certain major historic events, such as the settlement of the continent by the Europeans. The diseases they introduced were determined by the diseases present in their society in England and by the conditions under which they lived. On arrival in Australia, these diseases were transmitted to a people who had previously been sheltered from their effects, and spread under the influences of new environmental conditions linked to a social system introduced from Europe as well as to the conflict that almost inevitably developed between these races.[2]

From the arrival of the First Fleet in 1788, infectious diseases caused great hardship. A number of factors that encouraged the transmission of infectious diseases were inherent in a migrant society which attracted people from all corners of the world, and in which settlers were always on the move, pioneering the country or simply moving around the various settlements. The greater the degree of population movement between and within nations, the greater the ease with which infectious diseases can spread. The separation of Victoria from New South Wales in 1851 and the discovery of gold in the same year led to a dramatic expansion of the population of Victoria. In 1851 there were 77 345 people (the figure excludes Aborigines); by 1854 the population had reached 236 789, three years later in 1857 there were 410 776; and by the end of Victoria's first decade the population had expanded to well over half a million (540 322). This amounts to a roughly sevenfold increase in ten years. Imagine the entire present population of all of the other Australian States plus the population of New Zealand, arriving in Victoria over a decade, and one can start to get some idea of the pressures (and opportunities) that faced Victoria at this time. Not the least of these pressures related to the health of the community. Immigration on this scale placed huge, indeed intolerable, strains on the resources and facilities of Melbourne. Haggar has noted:

> It is not difficult to understand why a dramatic change took place in the health of the community when gold fever struck . . . Communities were not prepared for immigration on that scale, and consequently the needs of daily living— accommodation, food, water, sanitation and employment—were lacking . . . The town [Melbourne] was surrounded by 'cities of tents' where unemployment, vice, starvation, disease and death abounded.[3]

In 1851 even the major streets in Melbourne were unstable and unsafe, subject to the vagaries of the weather and the impacts of livestock and vehicles. There was no underground drainage system for rainwater, and even sewage was carried away in open gutters; little bridges enabled people to cross these primitive sanitation trenches. It was not unknown for Melburnians to drown when rain caused the major streets to flood.[4] Writing in November 1852, a possibly somewhat biased commentator (a resident of Sydney) wrote that 'nowhere in the southern hemisphere does chaos reign so triumphant as in Melbourne' and argued that in his opinion 'a worse governed, worse drained, worse lighted, worse watered town of note is not on the face of the globe'.[5] The difficulties experienced by Melbourne during those early gold rush days, and in particular the health problems and the prevalence of infectious diseases, might lead one to suggest that the term usually applied to the psychological atmosphere of the period—gold fever—might well have been true in a medical sense.

It has been noted that 'Wherever gold was discovered, and people massed to the diggings, infectious diseases broke out . . . conditions and occupational hazards took their toll. The miners had little immunity when their settlements were swept with infectious diseases.'[6] Measles and related respiratory complications, for example, first recorded in Victoria in 1850, caused the deaths of many hundreds of children. Diphtheria (frequently confused with quinsy or croup), was first recorded in Victoria in 1858, yet by 1869, 4574 deaths had been reported—a shocking figure, even if one accepts that a good many supposed diphtheria victims in fact suffered from other ailments. Haggar states the problem concisely: 'Between 1861 and 1871 the birth rate rapidly increased as the young adult immigrants became parents, and consequently there was a disastrous death rate among children from measles, scarlet fever, whooping-cough and diphtheria'.[7] Describing the impact of infectious diseases in Melbourne, Barrett noted in his study of the evolution of Melbourne's inner suburbs that 'During the nineteenth century, Australia was continually threatened by 'zymotic' [i.e. acute infectious] diseases—diarrhoea, dysentery, typhus-like fevers, scarlet fever, diphtheria, measles and smallpox. In Victoria in 1854–62 these diseases caused between a quarter and a half of all deaths each year.'[8] In a 'good' year, infectious diseases accounted for one in four of all deaths; in a 'bad' year—when some form of epidemic occurred—this rose to one in two of all deaths. Dramatic as these figures are, they do not tell the full tale because they disguise the fact that children constituted a large proportion of the victims of infectious disease. It was, of course, impossible to make any real progress in fighting infectious diseases until an accurate analysis of the causes of infection could be arrived at. Barrett describes this process in Melbourne:

> Before the impact of bacteriology in the 1800s, the most influential conception of disease in Australia, as elsewhere, was the 'miasmatic' one. According to this, disease was caused . . . by bad air (as in 'mal–aria'). Even when the disease was recognised as being communicable from person to person (e.g., plague, leprosy

and smallpox), the 'contagion' was conceived as chemical (a vapour or miasma emanating from the patient or from his wounds), not as biological. In most diseases common in Victoria, person-to-person contact was less obvious; here the ruling assumption was that the bad air emanated from filth in the environment—from swamps, stagnant pools, dirty rivers and accumulations of decomposing manure and garbage.[9]

The Central Board of Health had been set up by the government in 1855 to advise it and the municipalities on public health. The Board was a proponent of the miasma theory, and attributed disease spread to atmospheric causes like changes of temperature, east winds and impurities from stagnant water. In its report of 1859, it indirectly blamed bad drainage for many deaths from diphtheria, scarlet fever and measles.

As the nineteenth century progressed, people became less inclined to take a fatalistic attitude towards infectious disease and demands that 'something must be done' arose within the community. There was a great deal of debate over what that 'something' was. The fight against infectious disease was handicapped, indeed undermined, by the lack of understanding of its causes and mode of transmission. It is difficult for us today to appreciate the terrible grip that infectious diseases—typhoid, croup, whooping cough, diarrhoeal diseases and (to a lesser extent) measles and scarlatina—had on the community. The extent of the problem is seen in studies of the inner Melbourne suburb of Collingwood, which have shown that half of all deaths from infectious diseases were of infants under one year of age. The same suburb experienced an outbreak of the universally dreaded smallpox in 1884 and generally, as a poor and somewhat unhygienic suburb, was seen as being particularly susceptible to the two diseases which were associated in the public, and indeed the medical, mind with poor hygiene—typhoid and diphtheria, the so-called 'filth diseases'.

Diphtheria was such a severe health problem that the Victorian government in 1872 appointed a Royal Commission to inquire into all aspects of the disease. The state of medical knowledge and the worth of the completed report can be gleaned from one of the commissioner's main recommendations: 'We desire to record in the strongest possible manner our conviction of the absolute necessity of every householder in Victoria keeping a supply of sulphur in the house. Its fumes are the most powerful and valuable disinfectant we possess.'[10]

Mortality figures for Melbourne suggest that the two 'filth diseases' actually increased during the 1880s, peaking in 1890—twelve Collingwood residents died from typhoid in 1886, for example. Given these figures and its rather unsavoury reputation as a disease-ridden area, it is hardly surprising

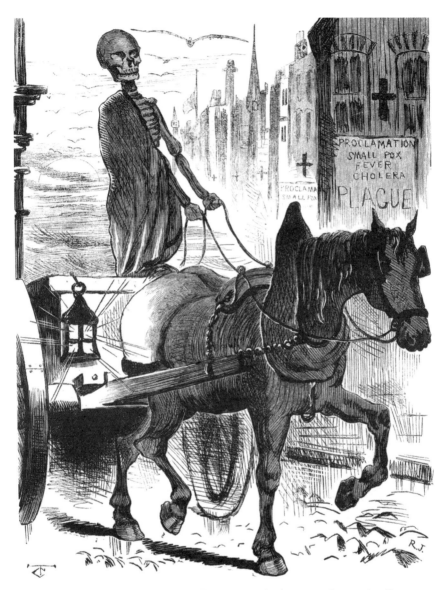

'Bring Out Your Dead', a grim cartoon from nineteenth-century Melbourne (Melbourne Punch, *21 January 1869*).

that Collingwood was one of the first municipalities to provide financial support to the Queen's Memorial Hospital.

Just as we have grown accustomed to the road toll, people in the nineteenth century had to some extent come to terms with the devastating effects of infectious diseases. A good example of this can be seen in the actual

Diphtheria was described in 1826 by Pierre Bretonneu, and the organism responsible, *Corynebacterium diphtheriae*, was isolated in 1883. Transmission is primarily by infected droplets and contamination from infected nasal discharge, but it can also be spread by contaminated milk. It is characterised by the formation of a membrane across the throat, causing breathing difficulties. Diphtheria appeared dramatically on an epidemic scale in Europe, America, Africa, China and the Pacific in 1858. Melbourne's first recorded death due to diphtheria occurred in October 1858, followed rapidly by others, and the death rate rose steadily until 1860. In 1859 antitoxin was first used in Australia, and in the 1920s an effective toxoid was produced. Subsequent widespread immunisation has greatly reduced the incidence of this once dreaded disease.

structure of families. One of the main reasons that large families were the order of the day was a recognition that the chances of children surviving to adulthood were not good; therefore parents took account of the likelihood of some of their children dying in infancy or early childhood when 'planning' the number of children they would have (it was also fairly common to name a number of boys in the one family with the traditional family first name in the hope that one of them would survive to carry on the name.)

The 'bad air' theory of disease transmission was gradually being superseded by new and more accurate theories on the spread of disease. Until about 1870 the miasmic theory was largely unchallenged in Australia (although it had long been recognised that diseases uncommon in Australia such as leprosy, plague, smallpox and cholera were contagious). In 1874 Dr William Thomson, a Melbourne medical practitioner, was arguing that typhoid fever, which was at the time a major scourge in Australia, was a contagious rather than miasmic disease. At this time the germ transmission theory of the spread of all infectious diseases was slowly becoming accepted. (Rejected by most Victorian doctors in the 1870s, it began to receive more general acceptance in the 1880s, even although many people still struggled to understand the concept). This new theory finally put to rest the miasmic theory of disease transmission, and it was realised that a disease like typhoid fever was not caused by bad air but by the ingestion of microscopic organisms —germs—originating in the excreta of someone infected by typhoid fever.

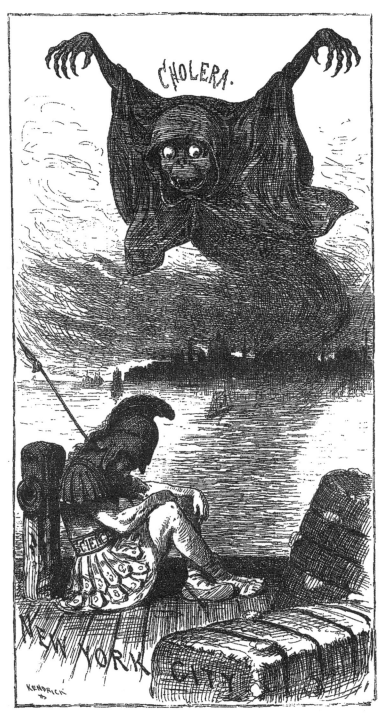

A nineteenth-century view of cholera

Smallpox (*Variola major, Variola minor*) has been described as 'the Most Dreadful Scourge of the Human Species'. It is a highly contagious viral disease, with symptoms including fever and skin eruptions that generally left pitted scars—pock marks—on the skin The name distinguishes it from 'great pox' (syphilis) which can cause major skin eruptions. Smallpox was first recorded in China in the fourth century CE and considered to have become endemic in populous areas of Asia and Europe by 1000 CE. The disease continued to be endemic in Europe until the development of a vaccine by Edward Jenner in about 1800.

While it seems likely that smallpox had been introduced to Aboriginal peoples by Macassan traders, there were severe epidemics after European settlement. Such an epidemic occurred among inland Aborigines in 1830 and spread widely throughout the country. From 1850 onwards the white settler community suffered many outbreaks (twenty-three separate outbreaks between 1850 and 1926). The Victorian outbreak of 1857 was introduced by the ship *Commander Perry*, docking at Melbourne, and the epidemic of 1868–69 by the *Avonvale*. An Act was passed in Victoria in 1854 making it compulsory for all babies to be vaccinated for smallpox before the age of six months. The legislation was amended in 1910 to incorporate a so-called 'conscience clause' (to allow parents to refuse vaccination). By the time the legislation was annulled in 1931, only 1 per cent of babies had been vaccinated in the preceding year. The story of smallpox has a triumphant ending—smallpox has been eliminated both in Australia and world wide, largely as a result of mass vaccination programs.

Although Victoria was perhaps a touch slow in accepting and acting on the latest advances in medical science, it cannot be faulted in terms of its willingness to introduce legislation on infectious diseases and other health matters. There was much health-related legislation prior to the opening of the hospital in 1904, reflecting the importance which health issues and infectious disease had in the community and highlighting the intense focus on attempts to control infectious diseases. The *Management of Towns Act* of 1854 contained 'sanitary provisions' to 'control the disposal of privy, cesspool, night-soil and other offensive matter'.

The first Act of the Victorian Parliament referring specifically to health was passed in 1855, 'for promoting the public health in populous places in the Colony of Victoria.' It created a Central Board of Health, and constituted every municipal council a Local Board of Health. It made provision for the appointment of medical officers of health by Local Boards, for the control of drains and sewers and for the seizure of unwholesome foods. It imposed upon all local authorities the duty of reporting to the Central Board the appearance of any epidemic or contagious disease. The Central Board was given power to issue directions and regulations to prevent epidemic diseases. (The Act was an almost exact copy of the *English Public Health Act* of 1848.) In 1857 a special Act—to remain operative for one year—was passed as a result of an epidemic of smallpox. This Act required medical practitioners and householders to report all smallpox cases.

The *Consolidation Act / Public Health Act* of 1865 brought together all previous legislation. The *Public Health Act* detailed the functions and powers of the Central and Local Boards of Health and included sections dealing with food adulteration, lodging houses, pollution of the Yarra River, vaccination, quarantine and cemeteries. In 1876 the *Amending Public Health Act* extended existing powers relating to infectious diseases and in particular empowered local authorities to provide means for disinfection and ambulance transport to hospital for patients. The Act outlawed cesspools. (Sections were copied directly from the English *Public Health Act* of 1875.) This was followed in 1878 by the *Conservation of Public Health Act*. The *Amending Health Act* of 1883 extended the 1865 Act and placed legal responsibility on medical practitioners to notify the occupier of the house of any case of smallpox, plague, cholera, yellow fever or other malignant infectious or contagious disease. The occupier, in turn, was obliged to inform the Local Board of Health.

The *Public Health Act* of 1888 invested more complete control over Local Boards of Health to the Central Board of Health and made special provisions for medical practitioners reporting infectious diseases. This was amended in 1889 by the *Public Health Act Amendment Act*. This Act was designed to implement the recommendations of the Royal Commission on the Sanitary Condition of Melbourne. The Act abolished the Central Board of Health and established a Department of Public Health to replace it. A new Central Board of Health was established by the *Health Act* of 1890. Amending Health Acts were passed in 1894, 1900 and 1903.

These legislative attempts to tackle the problems of infectious disease were spurred by publications that highlighted sanitary and other health problems and urged the government to introduce changes. The titles of some of these books and reports published in Melbourne tell their own sad story—

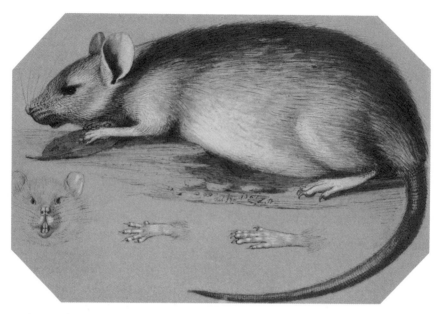

Ludwig Becker, artist and naturalist, who was to die during the Burke and Wills expedition, recorded the long-haired or plague rat in pen and ink and watercolour in 1861 (Ludwig Becker Sketchbook).

What Kills Our Babies, On the Excessive Mortality of Infants (1859); *Sanitary Conditions in Melbourne* (1868); *Dirt and Disease* (1872); *On the Advantages of Burning the Dead* (1873); *What Shall We Do With Our Dead* (1878); *Typhoid Fever in Victoria* (1883); *Report on Sewerage of Melbourne* (1890). These and many other books, pamphlets, lectures and newspaper articles not only reflected public concern, indeed public fears, but also helped to lead Victoria towards initiating steps to fight infectious diseases.

A number of other factors combined to provide the impetus for the establishment of the state's first infectious diseases hospital. In 1874, the Central Board of Health, in presenting to the government its fifteenth report (the first had been eighteen years earlier) said:

> As far back as the beginning of 1869 we recommended to the government the erection of an hospital, in the vicinity of the metropolis, for the isolation and treatment of contagious or infectious diseases which may, at any time, be introduced to the colony by an evasion of the quarantine laws which it is not possible at all times to prevent, and such has already, in fact occurred, as for instance in the Smallpox invasions of 1857 and 1869. We found it necessary to urge this matter on the government from time to time before anything was done, but we

are glad now to be able to mention the fact lately communicated to us by your directions, that provision be made for this object on the Estimates of the ensuing financial year.[11]

The Board went further than merely recommending the establishment of an infectious diseases hospital; it also commented on two sites which had been suggested as suitable and on the objections which had been, or might be, made to them. The two sites discussed were Royal Park (near the present Children's Hospital) and 'near Yarra Bend Asylum'. In responding to objections to the sites the Board rather disingenuously argued that the 'the objections which have been raised are more sentimental than founded on any real grounds of apprehension of danger . . . Although the existence of such provision is necessary . . . the necessity for the actual use of such an hospital is likely to but very rarely arise.'[12] This was a pointless, circuitous argument: either the facility was required or it was not required; one cannot argue for the construction of a hospital on the grounds that it is not in fact needed!

Royal Park does not appear to have remained under serious consideration for long, and the Yarra Bend site remained the favoured spot for an infectious diseases hospital. The Yarra Bend site, which is today Yarra Bend National Park, was originally part of Jika Jika Parish and was withheld from the parish's land sales in 1840. A 'Lunatic Asylum' was built on part of the site in 1848 and remained there until it was relocated across the river to Kew in 1880. The site then had the advantage of being owned by the government, being fairly near the centre of Melbourne yet relatively isolated, and having a tradition of being used for a health facility encompassing a custodial or near-custodial function. It is also worth mentioning that the site is one of great natural beauty

Within a few years of the Central Board of Health's Report, the Children's Hospital in Melbourne faced acute problems in coping with infectious diseases. A child admitted for other causes in 1877 contracted diphtheria after being treated in a ward which also housed patients suffering from diphtheria. The hospital committee made a number of responses to try to stop any future cross-infections occurring in the hospital. One sensible move was an improvement in ward ventilation, but from the perspective of the establishment of the Queen's Memorial Hospital the most important initiative was that the committee ruled that in future, unless they were obviously dying, children suffering from infectious diseases were not to be admitted. If patients already admitted to the hospital had the misfortune to catch an infectious disease, the committee decreed that such patients were to be transferred to a specially constructed wooden structure built in 1878 known as 'The Pavilion', where an 'Infectious Nurse' would be isolated with the patients.

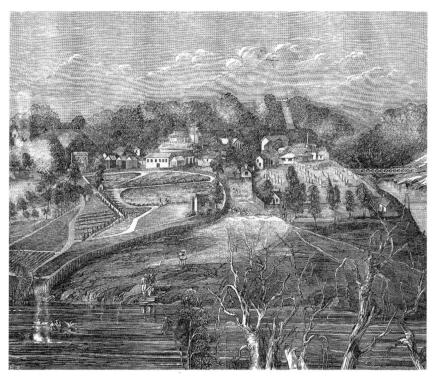

A wood engraving by Frederick Gross of the Yarra Bend Asylum for the Insane, 1868.

Although the Children's Hospital had taken sensible steps to reduce and contain problems relating to infectious diseases, it had not, of course, taken any positive steps to provide care and treatment for children suffering from infectious diseases—indeed its main thrust was to exclude such unfortunates. That this was no minor problem is demonstrated by the fact that by 1890 the Children's Hospital was turning away more than twenty cases of typhoid fever each week. Even though very few patients suffering from infectious diseases were knowingly admitted to the Children's Hospital, nurses at the hospital continued to die each year as a result of infections transmitted from patients, and there was a continuing problem of cross-infection among outpatients. Because of concern regarding the infectious potential of outpatients, the hospital issued each outpatient who displayed suspicious symptoms with a 'red for danger' ticket and transferred them to an area of the hospital reserved for infectious disease patients under the care of an 'Infectious Outpatients Nurse'.

One of Melbourne's other major public hospitals, the Alfred Hospital, had responded to the problems of caring for patients suffering from infectious diseases by erecting a tent in the hospital grounds, but the Board of Health

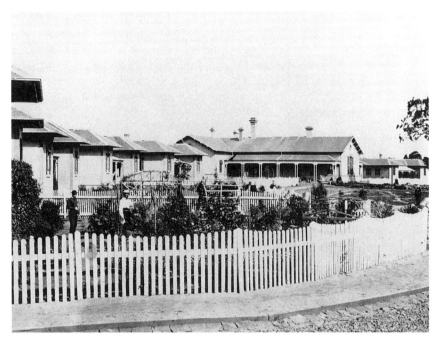

Cottages at the Yarra Bend Asylum, photographed in about 1861.

discouraged this type of initiative and refused a request from the Children's
Hospital Committee when they canvassed the Board for permission to follow
the lead of the Alfred Hospital and erect an infectious diseases tent or ward.

One of the most important and far-reaching publications on health
conditions in Melbourne was Gresswell's *Report of the Sanitary Condition of
Melbourne*, published in four parts in Melbourne in 1890. Dr Dan Astley
Gresswell, health officer of the City of Melbourne and later chair of the
Board of Public Health, stressed the desperate need for an infectious diseases hospital in Melbourne, basing his argument, in part, on the success of
the Belvedere Fever Hospital in Glasgow (which he described as being 'one
of the most perfect institutions of the kind'). The publication of Gresswell's
report has been seen as marking the real birth of Queen's Memorial Hospital,
although, as we have seen, the Central Board of Health had recommended a
contagious diseases hospital as early as 1869. In a paper on the history of
Fairfield hospital, Sandland has drawn attention to Gresswell's role in the
establishment of the hospital:

> He argued for a large central institution, rather than several small ones 'even if
> many of the patients have to be conveyed a considerable distance, this need not
> be regarded as important, as comfortable ambulance waggons would of course

be provided.' Later the philosophy of the era is emphasised: 'The principle at the foundation of such institutions, as compared with general hospitals, is that the isolation of the patient is carried out, not so much for his benefit as in the interests of the general public, by whom the expenses are rightly borne.' This meant that when the hospital was founded it was free to the patients, and a number of councils increasing over the early years contributed from their rates to the hospital's running costs.[13]

Lack of funding for the building of an infectious diseases hospital delayed the construction of this much-needed facility for over a quarter of a century, and certainly proved to be a much more intransigent problem than finding a suitable site. Eventually an opportunity arose in 1897 through Queen Victoria's Diamond Jubilee Fund. The Queen stipulated that any funds raised throughout the Empire to celebrate her 60-year reign were to be used 'towards the amelioration of the sick and suffering of the community'. At the suggestion of the Governor of Victoria, Lord Brassey, the Mayor of Melbourne, Councillor Strong, convened a meeting in Melbourne to discuss the establishment of a fever hospital. As the general and specialist hospitals in Melbourne had demonstrably failed to cope with the severe and recurrent demands made on their resources by infectious diseases such as typhoid and

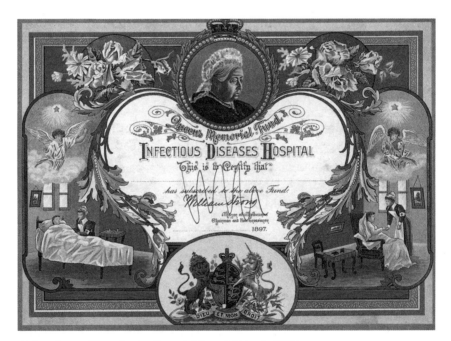

A donation certificate for the Queen's Memorial Fund, 1897.

diphtheria—and indeed had often simply refused to admit infectious disease patients as a matter of policy—it is hardly surprising that this meeting greeted the proposal to establish a 'Fever Hospital' enthusiastically. A fund-raising committee was immediately set up. This committee comprised representatives from the municipalities of Boroondara, Brighton, Brunswick, Essendon, Flemington and Kensington, Footscray, Hawthorn, Heidelberg, Kew, North Melbourne, Malvern, Northcote, Prahran, South Melbourne, St Kilda and Williamstown. Subscribers to the fund were told that all the money raised would be spent on the construction of a fever hospital, and that if enough money was raised the buildings would be completed in 1901.

The Queen's Memorial Fund Committee organised concerts and other activities. One notable aspect of the campaign was a specially written 'heart rending' poem published in the *Argus* on 17 April 1897 (the poem was also widely circulated in Melbourne as a fund-raising appeal flyer). The poem made an unashamedly emotional appeal for contributions:

The Cry of the Fever-Stricken Ones
by 'Oriel'

Hark to that cry, like a strange distant warning
That comes when the starlight melts out of the sky,
'Twixt the death of the night and the birth of the morning,
When Nature's at ebb, and sick people die!
Listen once for it! Can you not hear it?
It rises, it sinks to a whisper again;
Low as the voice of the sea, but as ceaseless—
The cry of the victims of sickness and pain

Shall we be deaf to that cry, or offended,
Careless of brotherhood, careful of gold,
Leaving the flickering lantern untended,
Till at last it dies out in the cold?
Think of it, you who have found the sweet secret,
Felt how love's flame can transfigure life's clay,
Somebody's lover or somebody's sweetheart.
Helpless among us, is dying today

Yes and the children! The children resemble
The clustering stars in the long summer night;
At times in the heavens above us they tremble,
And soften the roughness of Earth with their light.
But sometimes, in summer, all round the horizon
The stars fall in showers, their bright starry life
Flashing out in a moment from light into darkness—
And so fall the children when sickness is rife.

Can you, conceiving mere greed as a pleasure,
So hold to the bitter, abandon the sweet;
Piling up silver and gold without measure,
But treading the daisies down under your feet?
Yet long ago it was promised by Someone,
Who lovingly, help for the children implored,
That if only you gave one a cup of cold water,
You surely in no wise should lose your reward!

So, happily remembering the fountain of tresses,
The glad sunny eyes and cheeks all a-glow
The frank, open laughter and joyous caresses,
Of one who has gone where the roses all go.
You may think of these children by fever tormented,
Babies distraught and delirious with pain,
Asking in whispers, for just a cool pillow,
Asking for help—shall they ask in vain?

Although lachrymose, even sickly, by today's standards and tastes, Oriel's poem certainly spoke directly to Victorian sentimentality; more importantly, it touched on the very real problem of the large number of children who died as a result of infectious diseases. Oriel's children did not 'ask in vain'. For such a good cause, and one that moreover was a homage to Queen Victoria, Victorians were prepared to dig deep and, by 1897, £16 000 had been raised. To have raised such a substantial sum in such a short space of time reflected great credit upon the organisers of the appeal and the generosity of the Victorian public. It also reflected the fact that the community was acutely aware of the desperate need for a specialised infectious diseases hospital. In April 1898 the state government provided very welcome support to the project when it officially set aside 15 acres of the Yarra Bend site and called for designs to build a fever hospital.

A perspective had been prepared by architects Wharton Down and Gibbons in 1893, showing a proposed infectious diseases hospital for Melbourne, and this may have helped the architects chosen to design the hospital buildings—Clegg, Kell and Miller, a Ballarat company—in preparing their design. The hospital was built by the building contractor, R. Stockdale. When completed, the hospital stood on a 22-acre site and comprised two wards, for scarlet fever and diphtheria respectively, an administration block, kitchen, laundry, receiving house, lodge and nurses' home (with accommodation for twenty nurses). The two wards each contained twenty-five beds, were well ventilated and were floored with bitumen (for ease of cleaning). Asphalt paths linked the various buildings, and the kitchen block was situated at the centre of the whole complex. The hospital was designed to be a 'locked' facility (an

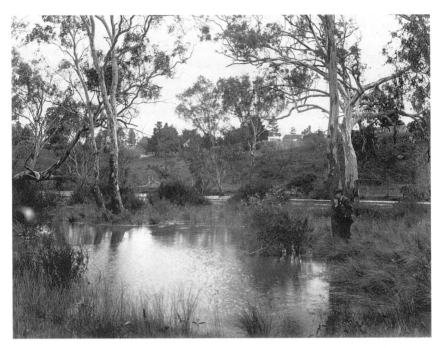

The Yarra River at Fairfield in 1901, close to land set aside in 1898 to build a fever hospital.

infectious diseases hospital has a custodial role as well a caring role). Access to and from the hospital was controlled by resident lodge-keepers, and there were separate entries for infected and non-infected traffic. These hospital buildings have been described by an architectural historian: 'Externally the first buildings were of a cavity face-brickwork with stucco dressings and Marseilles pattern terra-cotta tiles; they generally followed the Queen Anne or Federation style of architecture'.[14] The two original wards were 'characterised by two conically roofed octagonal tower rooms on the north end, presumably acting as service rooms for the staff. The balance of the building being a long, hipped roof and verandahed pavilion, which illustrates the Oriental aspects of this style of architecture.'[15] Entry to the new hospital was by a private drive leading to Yarra Bend Asylum, from which visitors entered the hospital grounds. A *Weekly Times* journalist described the hospital at its opening as being an enclosure 'in which several substantial looking buildings stand at respectful distances from one another, in a bare uncultivated allotment of twenty-two acres'.[16]

The hospital was completed in 1901, the year of Queen Victoria's death. It was not opened until October 1904 (35 years after the original Board of

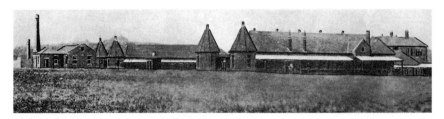

The new hospital, in 1904 (from the Golden Jubilee Brochure).

Health discussions) due to a lack of funds—the Queen's Memorial Fund having been exhausted in paying for the building of the hospital, no money was forthcoming for furniture, supplies or staffing. The first meeting of the hospital's Committee of Management was held on 16 May 1904 at Melbourne Town Hall. Melbourne Councillor Sir M. D. McEacharn was elected chair, and committee members were councillors and aldermen from Melbourne, Fitzroy, Richmond, St. Kilda, Brunswick and Coburg. Five members had to retire each year, and the first meeting drew lots to decide upon the order of retirement. Four sub-committees were set up—Furnishing and Equipment; House and Building; Finance; and Staff—the chair being an ex officio member of all four.[17] In terms of the actual conduct of the hospital's pre-opening business, it was 'arranged that for the time being the business of the Institution be conducted by the Melbourne City Council pending the appointment of permanent officers,' and that McEacharn act as honorary treasurer pending the appointment of a treasurer. Although the hospital had been vacant since the buildings were completed in 1901, it had already fallen into debt of £188 18s 1d, incurred 'principally in payment of wages to care-taker, insurance, and other expenses'. The Committee agreed to make good the deficiency 'under the circumstances'. The first task facing the newly formed Committee was to make all the preparations necessary to provide the furnishings, equipment, staffing and provisions which were required to turn the bare hospital buildings into a functional hospital, This was to prove no mean task.

The Furnishing and Equipment Sub-committee met on 18 May and appointed Alderman Strong as committee chair. It decided that 'as far as practicable tenders would be invited for the various supplies required by the Hospital according to samples to be exhibited by the Committee'. It was also decided to 'ask the authorities of the Melbourne Hospital to favour the Committee ... with samples of the various articles supplied to that Institution'. This was the first of many instances in which the new hospital

Committee of Management and the various sub-committees would seek assistance from the long-established and respected Melbourne Hospital (Royal Melbourne Hospital) in that months that followed. It is pleasing to note that the men entrusted with establishing the hospital were not too proud to seek the assistance of knowledgeable people and that the Melbourne Hospital gave unstintingly. This meeting made speedy, one might even say urgent, arrangements for the whole Committee of Management to inspect the new hospital buildings the following day—some, perhaps all, of them may never have seen the buildings before. The Furnishing and Equipment Sub-committee visited the Melbourne Hospital the day after, to see at first hand how a hospital was furnished and equipped. The 'Lady Superintendent' of the Melbourne Hospital had already helped prepare a list of articles that the new hospital would need for the Queen's Memorial Fund Committee, and she discussed this list with the sub-committee during their visit.

The Committee of Management and its various sub-committees worked hard over the following months to prepare the new hospital for opening. The minutiae of their efforts need not detain us here but we should note the huge amount of work, much of which was unfamiliar to the committee members, who mostly lacked experience in hospital administration and medical matters. The first major decision of the Committee of Management was taken on 26 May, when it resolved to advertise for a Medical Superintendent and a Matron. The Medical Superintendent would receive £200 per annum with full board and lodgings, and the Matron £80, also with full board and lodgings. Given that the hospital had been sitting unused for three years, the Committee of Management wisely delegated the House and Buildings Sub-committee to prepare a report on the repairs that would be required to the hospital buildings.

The Finance Sub-Committee met for the first time on 30 May and immediately faced the problem of how to finance the opening of the hospital. The Queen's Memorial Fund monies had been completely spent and an overdraft of £44 10s 6d had been drawn. The Finance Sub-committee decided to recommend to the Committee of Management that a levy of £1500 be made upon the municipalities for furnishing and equipping the hospital and for expenses which would inevitably arise prior to the receipt of the first quarterly contributions from councils. The sub-committee also authorised the town clerk to apply to the hospital's bank (Bank of Australia) for a £500 overdraft. The Committee of Management accepted all of the Finance Sub-committee's recommendations.

A special sub-committee met on 7 June to discuss government conditions relating to the hospital. It examined a number of conditions which had caused some concern and found that it was able to accept them. Included in these conditions were the total enclosure of the hospital site by a 'high iron fence'; the prohibition on admitting cases of smallpox, plague or other exotic diseases, and annual payment of the government contribution to the hospital. The fact that the hospital was to be restricted to treating patients suffering from scarlet fever and diphtheria was to be a continuing problem for the hospital in its early years.

At the Committee of Management meeting held on 9 June 1904, the main item on the agenda was the responses to the advertisement for a Medical Superintendent and a Matron. The response had in fact been rather patchy: while eleven women had applied for the Matron's position, only one application was received for the Medical Superintendent. A short list of people to be interviewed was decided upon for the Matron's job, and a very short list consisting of one man for the Medical Superintendent's job. At the next meeting of the Committee of Management, on 16 June, it was resolved to appoint Dr Sydney H. Allen FRCSB as the hospital's first Medical Superintendent and Miss E. A. Conyers as the first Matron. Both engagements were to begin on 20 June. The Furnishing Sub-committee, which met on that day, not surprisingly decided to 'at once obtain the furniture necessary for the offices of the Medical Superintendent and the Matron'. This meeting had the pleasant task of responding to an offer by the Australian Natives' Association of £75 towards the purchase of an ambulance. Given the financial difficulties the committee was facing, such an offer was welcome indeed.

Scarlet fever (Scarlatina) is an acute infectious disease, especially prevalent among children. Caused by haemolytic streptococci, the disease is characterised by a bright red rash spreading from the upper to the lower part of the body (hence the name) and a sore throat. The rash is followed by the skin peeling in flakes—the disease thus echoing the effects of severe sunburn. Daniel Sennert, a German physician, is credited with the first description of scarlet fever in 1617. It was frequently confused with measles. Scarlet fever was apparently unknown in Australia till 1833. It was recorded in and around Melbourne in 1841, and reappeared with greater severity in 1848. There were subsequently irregular epidemics, declining in importance from 1880 onwards. Scarlet fever can now be successfully treated with antibiotics.

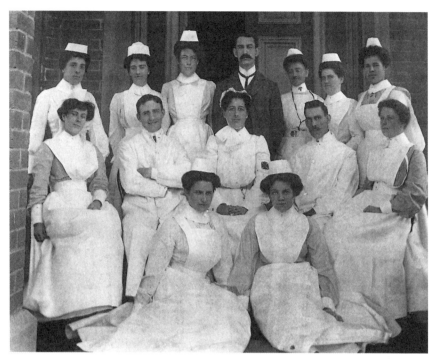

In the second row of the staff for the new hospital, 1904, are Dr S. H. Allen, Medical Superintendent (left) and Miss E. A. Conyers, Matron (centre).

The next meeting of the Committee of Management, on 23 June, considered the thorny subject of what classes of diseases should be admitted to the hospital at its opening. The Medical Superintendent reported that two classes of disease could be treated at the same time, given the existing accommodation. After further deliberation it was decided that only cases of scarlet fever and diphtheria be admitted to the hospital. This meeting also decided to erect a porter's lodge at the main entrance to the hospital (at a cost not exceeding £20). The question of staffing was much discussed at this meeting, and it was decided to ask the Medical Superintendent and the Matron to advise regarding the hospital's staffing requirements and to ask the town clerk to obtain particulars as to wages paid to staffs at other hospitals in Melbourne. A special Committee of Management meeting was arranged for 27 June to consider the whole issue of staffing and wages.

In keeping with its role as Melbourne's newest and most modern hospital, the committee decided that the hospital should be connected with the central telephone exchange and that quotations should be invited for the installation of a 'complete telephonette' service between the various hospital buildings. Another important development at this meeting was the tabling of a plan for laying out and planting the hospital grounds by Guilfoyle and Campbell. The committee accepted the report and decided to ask for a further report from the same firm regarding how the work should be scheduled and what trees should be purchased first.

At the special Committee of Management meeting held on 27 June, the Medical Superintendent and Matron reported that in their opinion the nursing and domestic staff required by the hospital at its capacity of fifty patients was fourteen nursing staff (2 sisters, 3 night nurses and 9 nurses), ten domestic staff (2 wardsmaids, 1 maid for domestic block, 1 maid for nursing home, 1 cook and 2 assistants, 1 laundress and 2 assistants) and six men (1 ambulance driver, 2 porters, 2 engine drivers and 1 disinfector). The committee accepted this estimate that the hospital would require thirty staff to operate, and set up a sub-committee to recommend a scale of wages to be paid to the various staff members. This sub-committee met on 30 June and after considering the rates paid in other comparable institutions recommended that the following pay scales be adopted by the hospital: sisters, £40 per annum; nurses, £30 per annum; probationer nurses (1st year) £12, (2nd year) £18, (3rd year) £24; ward and housemaids, 10s per week; laundress, 16s per week (this works out at £40 per annum—the same wage as a sister); assistant laundress, 10s per week; cook (female), 20s per week (£52 per annum!); assistant cooks, 10s per week; engine drivers (resident), £9 per month, (non-resident— the senior officer) £12 per month; disinfector, 20s per week, ambulance driver, 20s per week and porters, 16s per week. All of these staff were also to be provided with board and residence, with the exception of the non-resident senior engine driver. The relativities between the salaries of the various types of staff make fascinating reading, highlighting as it does the extreme nature of gender inequalities and the lowly respect—at least in terms of financial remuneration—accorded to nursing staff. The Committee of Management accepted the salary recommendations at a meeting held on 30 June. This meeting also decided that the time had arrived to advertise at once for 'Sisters, nurses and such others are immediately required'. The meeting went on to consider applications received for the two nursing sister positions and decided to employ M. J. Young and E. M. Groves. The task of selecting other nurses and ancillary staff was delegated to the Medical Superintendent and the Matron. A special sub-committee was set up to select the six male employees required.

Even although the Committee of Management had reached an advanced stage in preparing for the opening of the hospital, a number of important building issues still needed to be addressed and two new building projects were approved. The first was the decision to call for the preparation of plans for a two-stall stable with feed and harness room and an ambulance car shed. The second building decision arose from an inspection of the hospital made by Cr Stapley, a member of the House and Building Sub-committee. Stapley, who clearly had some knowledge of building design, reported to the Committee of Management that it was 'absolutely essential that verandahs should be erected along the west side [of the two wards] and submitted an offer by Mr. R. Stockdale, contractor for the erection of the buildings, to erect such verandahs at a cost of £74 each'. It is greatly to the credit of the Committee of Management that, when they were incredibly busy with the myriad arrangements which had to be made prior to opening the hospital, they still found the time—and the money—to discuss and approve a fairly substantial addition to the hospital's buildings. Many thousands of patients and staff had reason to thank the wisdom and foresight of Cr Stapley and his fellow committee members over the decades that followed as the verandahs provided them with great physical and aesthetic pleasure.

Turning empty buildings into a fully staffed, equipped and provisioned hospital is a task of Herculean proportions, and the various committees involved in the process had a welter of decisions and arrangement to make. At the Committee of Management meeting on 14 July, for example, the committee had to examine tenders presented for the supply of groceries (one year's supply), furniture, instrument tables, bedsteads, uniform samples, filters and sterilisers, laundry equipment, and wines and spirits, and select the most suitable offers. It also had to approve a contract for painting the hospital and the appointment of engine drivers, porters, a cook and a laundress. Adding to their worries, the Medical Superintendent and Matron rather surprisingly informed the committee that none of the applicants for nursing positions were considered suitable and that the positions would have to be re-advertised.

Major decisions regarding the hospital grounds were made at the meeting of the House and Buildings Sub-committee. Campbell and Guilfoyle Co. had recommended that elm, plane and poplar trees be planted to form the avenues along the walks and roads. After considering this expert advice the sub-committee decided to plant plane trees along the roadways and pepper trees in the grounds for shelter purposes. These decisions, made under pressure and amidst numerous other more pressing concerns, were sound and had a considerable impact on the aesthetic quality of the hospital in the years ahead.

The Committee of Management meeting held on 21 July noted that Sir Malcolm McEacharn the chair and honorary treasurer, had returned to Britain and that Alderman Strong had been authorised to sign cheques on the hospi-

tal account. A note from the town clerk tabled on 28 July noted the resignation of Sir Malcolm McEacharn and that he was to be replaced on the
committee by Cr W. W. Cabena. Cr Strong was elected chair in McEacharn's
place and was also appointed honorary treasurer. Given the difficulties in
attracting suitable applicants, the committee decided to increase the wage
offered to nurses from £30 per annum to £40 (to maintain salary relativities,
the salary of sisters was raised to £50 per annum). The committee also agreed
to employ M. Dwyer to perform clerical work at a salary of £2 10s per week,
a figure that dwarfs even the newly increased salaries of nursing staff. The
committee were informed that three pupil nurses (probationary) had been
taken on—Misses Sims, Willoby and Blackwood—and that the Royal Victorian Trained Nurses Association had been contacted regarding the require-
ment that the hospital be recognised by the association as a training hospital
for infectious diseases. The committee also agreed to send a letter of appreciation to the secretary and Lady Superintendent of Melbourne Hospital for
services rendered to the committee while it was equipping the hospital. The
meeting is notable in that it approved the following draft rules for nursing
staff (and incorporated rules for patients). These rules remained in place substantially unaltered for many, many years. Some are worth quoting, as they
provide a wonderful insight into the way the hospital operated and the living
and working conditions of both staff and patients:

Queen's Memorial Infectious Diseases Hospital
Rules Relating To Patients. Adopted 22 September, 1904.

1. Only such patients as are infected with or suffering from scarlet fever or
    diphtheria, or such other infectious diseases as may be specified from time
    to time by the Committee of Management shall be admitted to the
    Hospital . . .
3. Patients residing in any municipal district represented on the Committee of
    Management must furnish an order for admission signed by the Municipal
    Clerk or Officer of Health of such district.
4. Patients residing in any municipal district not represented on the Com-
    mittee of Management must furnish an undertaking to pay the cost of
    maintenance and treatment of such patients in the hospital. Such under-
    taking must be signed by the Municipal Clerk of such district on behalf of
    the Council of the district.
5. Patients from 'overseas' must furnish an order for admission signed by an
    Officer of the Board of Public Health . . .
7. Wherever practicable patients shall leave all valuables, money, &c., and all
    outside clothing, at home, and should wear body linen only, and be wrapped
    in blankets sent with the ambulance.

8. Every patient on arrival at the Hospital will be examined in the Receiving House, and if found to be infected with, or suffering from one of the infectious diseases mentioned in clause 1, will be admitted into the Ward set apart for treatment of such disease.

9. The clothes worn by the patient, and all other articles in his possession at the time of his admission shall be forthwith disinfected, and stored for the patient as may be directed by the Medical Superintendent. In cases where the clothes or other articles are of such a character as to render their destruction necessary, they may be destroyed, and a record thereof shall be duly made and preserved; but the Committee will not make any compensation for such articles . . .

10. The patients shall be dieted in such a manner, and at such times as the Medical Superintendent shall direct.

11. Patients admitted to the Hospital will be required to confirm to the following rules:–

   (a) They shall in all matters be subject to the control of the Medical Superintendent, or of the Matron or other members of staff acting under his instructions, and shall be respectful and obedient to the nurses.

   (b) They shall preserve silence during the night, and during the visit of the Medical Officers or Matron, and at all times refrain from making any noise which would disturb the other patients in the Ward.

   (c) They shall not leave their beds or the Ward without permission, and shall not enter any Ward except that to which they have been allotted, nor the nurses' duty room except by permission of the Ward Sister.

   (d) They shall, when in the grounds, confine themselves strictly to that portion thereof set apart for them, and shall not leave the grounds, nor communicate directly with any person outside the premises until discharged from the Hospital.

   (e) They shall retire to bed not later than 8 o'clock p.m., and shall at no time be absent from the Ward after dusk without leave.

   (f) They shall not send letters or parcels to anyone outside the Hospital, except in such cases of urgency, and then only by special permission of the Medical Superintendent or Matron. The letters or parcels in such cases must be given to the Ward Sister for purposes of disinfection. The Matron will always convey any message of urgency.

   (g) No visitors will be allowed to see patients except by special permission of the Medical Superintendent or Matron, and subject to the special rules relating thereto.

   (h) Patients shall not give anything to or receive anything from visitors except through the Medical Superintendent or Matron.

   (i) They shall not give any present or gratuity to any nurse or other official.

   (j) They shall, if able to do so, regularly wash themselves as required, and keep themselves scrupulously clean.

   (k) They shall remain in the Hospital so long as the Medical Superintendent thinks proper.

(l) All complaints must be made to the Medical Superintendent or Matron [scored out in red pen and replaced by secretary—in copy attached to the minutes] within three days from the occurrence of the cause for complaint . . .

13. Should any patient desire, or the parents or guardians of any patient, to be visited by a Minister of religion for the purpose of affording religious instruction or consolation, permission for such visit will be given, subject to such conditions as may be laid down by the Medical Superintendent in each case, but such instruction or consolation shall be given in such a way as not to interfere with the good order and discipline of the Hospital . . .

15. Notice of admission and discharge of each patient shall be sent to the Municipal Clerk of the district in which the patient resided at the time of admission.

16. On the occurrence of the death of a patient notice thereof will be at once sent to the nearest known relative or the guardian of such patient, and the body must be removed from the Hospital for internment within 24 hours from the time of death . . .

17. A charge of 4s.6d [handwritten in red:'4/6 subsequently altered to 7/6 September 1905—decided at a Comm of Man. meeting 31 Aug. 1905'] will be made for the treatment of each patient received into the Hospital for every day, or part of a day, during which the patient is in the Hospital.

18. In the event of a patient being brought to the Hospital by the Hospital Ambulance, who upon examination is found not to be infected with or suffering from one of the infectious diseases admissible to this Hospital, a charge of 3s per hour, or part of an hour, for the services of the ambulance and attendants will be made upon the person or Council at whose request the ambulance shall have been sent.

Having established staff and patient rules to cover almost all foreseeable contingencies, the Committee of Management on 8 September 1904 made the momentous decision to open the hospital on 1 October, and informed nursing staff that they were to present themselves for duty on Monday, 26 September, to prepare for the opening. At the last meeting before the opening, held on 23 September, the committee decided to appoint G. V. Silvester to the important position of Hospital Secretary and Steward. There were a number of last-minute problems. The town clerk, for example, informed the committee that they were still awaiting the ambulance promised by the Australian Natives' Association and that he had invited quotations from coachbuilders and livery stable proprietors for the temporary supply of a suitable conveyance to serve as an ambulance. On a lighter note the committee decided to hang a portrait of the late Queen—Her Majesty Queen Victoria—which had been presented to the hospital, on the western wall of the hall in the administrative block. It was obviously considered

appropriate that the good Queen should be allowed to watch over the operations of the hospital that had been designed as her memorial.

The hospital was inspected by members of the metropolitan councils on
Thursday, 29 September and opened on schedule on 1 October 1904. The
somewhat dubious honour of being the hospital's first patient fell to a woman
named Elsie Lewis, suffering from scarlet fever.

The opening of the hospital did not, of course, mean an end to the
work of the Committee of Management and its various sub-committees. The
hospital was still lacking a number of crucial items—a horse to pull its yet
non-existent ambulance, for example. On 4 October, the Furnishing and
Equipment Sub-committee decided to give a horse, which was for sale at
£25, a trial pulling a hospital ambulance.

At the first Committee of Management meeting after the opening of
the hospital, on 6 October, the Matron reported that the cook had given
notice and left the hospital and that a housemaid had left without giving
notice—both had been replaced. Unfortunately these precipitate resignations
were the beginning of a pattern which was to become increasingly obvious in
the months ahead, reflecting some serious problems in relations between
senior staff and their junior charges. The Medical Superintendent reported

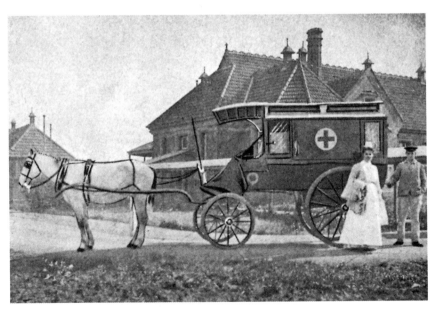

The hospital's first ambulance (from the Golden Jubilee Brochure).

that nine cases of scarlet fever and diphtheria had been admitted during the first week. This was less than 20 per cent bed occupancy, but this was not alarming at such an early stage in the hospital's life. The hospital still did not have its own ambulance. The Australian Natives' Association had not supplied the promised ambulance, as they were 'most anxious to provide the best article'. And two horses offered for sale as ambulance horses had not been purchased because the owners had failed to appear at arranged trials. The tale had a happy ending, however, as Cr Gardiner offered to lend the hospital a 'suitable horse for a week'. This kind offer was accepted with thanks.

Far more serious problems relating to the development, indeed to the very existence of the hospital as an independent institution, were already being encountered. These problems revolved around the hospital's admission policy and the related matter of hospital finances. For the first time the Committee of Management minutes showed serious divisions of opinion among committee members:

> The process of admission of patients into the Hospital was discussed. Alderman Burton stating that, as the Melbourne Hospital was the central Institution, it would be wise to act on the suggestion of the Medical Superintendent of that Hospital that he should be entrusted by the various municipalities with orders for admission ... Councillor Wheeler took exception to the remarks of Dr Moore at the recent meeting of the Melbourne Hospital Committee in referring to the building as a hideous mistake, and denounced the remarks as unjust and serious to the Hospital financially. It was eventually decided on the motion of Councillor McNair that circulars requesting the Municipalities to forward to the Medical Superintendent of the Melbourne Hospital signed orders for admission of patients to the Queen's Memorial Hospital.

At the Committee of Management meeting on 13 October the Medical Superintendent reported that six cases of scarlet fever and diphtheria had been admitted since 6 October and that one death had occurred. The death of this patient had become something of a public scandal and had caused the hospital a great deal of embarrassment and damage. The minutes note that:

> The reported delay in the admission of Beryl Beauchamp who died in the Hospital on Sunday last was investigated. Dr Wheeler complained that the facts of the case had been misstated in a section of the press, it having been made to appear that the patient had been taken to the Hospital gates, and refused admission, whereas the delay occurred before the patient was removed from her house and arose from the refusal of Northcote Town Clerk to at first issue the necessary guarantee. Dr Allen the Medical Superintendent explained that he had communicated with the Town Clerk of Northcote with the object of procuring the necessary documents for the immediate admission of the child, but no notice had been taken of his advice.

Although this explanation somewhat reduces the culpability of the hospital in the patient's death, there can be no doubt that, while the hospital was arguing with the town clerk of Northcote about who would pay the hospital treatment costs, a child was dying—this was one cry from a 'fever stricken one' which was not responded to in a truly caring and responsible fashion.

An invitation to the non-contributing councils to make satisfactory arrangements for the admission and financial support of patients to the Infectious Diseases Hospital had not met a positive response. Cr McNair gave notice that he would move at the next meeting 'That a deputation wait on the Honorary Premier to provide legislation giving power to this committee to enforce payments from the councils not contributing to the maintenance of the hospital for the treatment of patients from their respective districts'. (At the next meeting it was decided to defer this motion for a month while further negotiations took place with municipal councils regarding funding arrangements—militant political lobbying was not really the Committee of Management's forte.) Towards the end of the meeting the Medical Superintendent, for whom this must have been a rather difficult meeting, stated that under existing circumstances he could never leave the hospital and that he could not continue in the position unless he was given an assistant medical officer. The committee agreed that a recently qualified assistant medical officer be appointed on a six month contract with the possibility of extension for twelve months, and that an honorarium of £50 plus board and lodgings be allowed.

At last, on 20 October, it was reported at the House and Building Sub-committee meeting that the hospital had finally managed to buy a horse—a six-year-old at a cost of £27. Despite the delay the hospital could never be accused of having put the 'cart before the horse', as they were still without their own ambulance. On the same day, a Committee of Management meeting was informed by the Medical Superintendent that only six cases of scarlet fever and diphtheria had been admitted since 13 October. This level of admission was much lower than had been projected and was beginning to pose serious questions regarding the viability of the institution as a specialised infectious diseases hospital.

Staffing problems continued to concern the Committee of Management. On 27 October the Matron reported that a kitchen hand and a housemaid had left 'of their own accord' and that Effie McCoy, a wardsmaid, had been 'dismissed for disobedience', The large number of staff leaving the hospital was becoming almost as much of a worry as the small number of patient admissions. These concerns were to remain prominent over the following weeks. A kitchen hand, a cook, a kitchen maid, two wardsmaids, an assistant laundress, a nurse and the assistant medical officer had all left the hospital before the end of the year. It is fair to say that staff turnover—even for a new hospital—was unacceptably high.

Financial problems also continued to weigh heavily. By early December the Committee of Management had been forced to take a £750 overdraft (at $5\frac{1}{2}$ per cent interest) just to cover running costs. Responding to this financial situation, the Committee resolved on 8 December to approach the state government with a request that the hospital be given £1500 from 'Surplus Revenue'—perhaps hoping that the forthcoming season of goodwill might imbue the government with sufficient Christmas spirit to accede to the rather hopeful request. At this period the hospital's minute books start to record a good many sub-committee meetings being cancelled due to the lack of quorums. It appears that after the huge effort required to prepare the hospital for opening, some committee members started to lose interest in and enthusiasm for the project—feeling, no doubt, that they had 'done their bit' and that the hospital's paid employees should now shoulder the burden of running the hospital. When considering this development, which was to remain a problem for almost a decade, we should bear in mind that the members of the committee were extremely busy men for whom this task was but a small part of their duties as councillors and alderman, and that their voluntary work in local government was in turn secondary to their professional and business affairs. Small wonder then that, after the intense demands made upon their time and energies in the months leading up to the opening of the hospital, there was a tendency to rest on their laurels.

The Committee of Management made an inspection of the hospital on 12 January 1905. At its meeting the following week the main discussion revolved around whether the hospital should increase the daily rate for the treatment and maintenance of patients. Despite the urgent financial position of the hospital, the committee deferred a decision on this matter. On a related issue, the Medical Office asked the committee to consider admitting people suffering from 'some other class of disease', that is, from diseases other than scarlet fever and diphtheria. The Medical Superintendent was asked to make out a report for consideration. He presented his report to the Committee of Management on 2 February, recommending that, in view of the low average number of patients, additional infectious cases such as typhoid and septic diseases be admitted to the hospital. The report further stated that it would be necessary to appoint an honorary surgeon to be on call for serious cases. After some discussion the matter was referred to a sub-committee consisting of the chair and Crs Alexander and Wheeler. Attempting to tackle the problem from a different direction, Alexander placed on notice a motion regarding increasing the daily rate charged for hospital care. There was general agreement to this increase, but some problems were foreseen and it was decided that a decision on the matter be left for a month. The Matron, in what had become almost a hospital tradition, reported another staff 'movement': she had given the officers' house-maid a week's notice on account of inexperience. It is worth noting that this meeting decided to wait for three weeks before holding another meeting as this would 'suit the convenience of the members'. The meeting of the special sub-committee on the hospital's daily rate scheduled for 14 February had to be cancelled, as Alexander could not attend. The sub-committee, when it finally met three days later, decided against admitting patients suffering from diseases other than scarlet fever and diphtheria. It did, however, recommend that councils be 'urged to enforce the isolation of scarlet fever and diphtheria patients in their districts'.

Fairfield Hospital was not only the first infectious diseases hospital in Victoria, it was also purposely designed to undertake its specialised role. Dr Malcolm McEacharn (Associate Director of the American College of Surgeons), an international expert on hospitals and hospital design, who inspected the hospital in 1926, described it as the 'best fever hospital with which he had ever come in contact'.[18]

For well over thirty years after it first opened the hospital was supposed to take only patients with diseases gazetted as being treatable. At first, because of the public health priorities of the day, there were only two such diseases, diphtheria and scarlet fever. This selectivity in large part accounts for the fact that in its early years the hospital did not have to work to anything like its full capacity. In the eight months following the opening on 1 October 1904, only 313 patients were treated. The demands made on the resources of an infectious diseases hospital are, of course, unlike the demands made on general or even other specialised hospitals; they are completely unpredictable and perhaps best described as either 'drought or flood'. After an initial drought, a flood descended upon the hospital in 1909 when a scarlet fever epidemic swept through Melbourne. The hospital, which only had 50 beds, was treating up to 250 patients at any one time. Nursing staff (led by new Matron E. M. Walker, who was to remain Matron until her death in November 1938) were forced to stuff mattresses with straw to cope with the demand for beds, and the 23-year-old Medical Superintendent, Dr Gray, and his staff were working day and night. The extent of the problem can be seen by the fact that ten tents were erected to provide emergency temporary accommodation for the deluge of patients. It need hardly be said that these tents were unsuited to the vagaries of Melbourne's weather. Indeed one 'fierce autumn storm ripped through the temporary accommodation, calling attention to the want of proper facilities

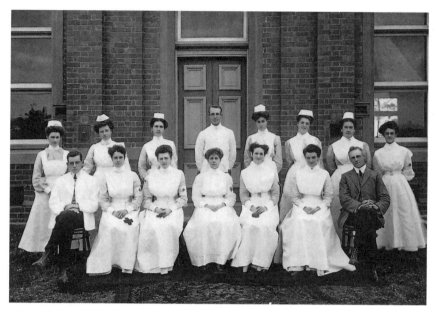

The staff in 1907: in the centre are Sr M. K. Moss, Medical Superintendent and Miss R. L. Sappere, Matron.

whenever Melbourne suffered an epidemic'.[19] These temporary facilities were still in use six years later when Dr Scholes, the Medical Superintendent, who replaced Gray in 1910, was forced to plead with the Board to install proper flooring in some of the still-functioning emergency tents.

In 1914 Anketell and his son Kingsley Henderson, two of Victoria's most prominent and influential hospital architects, took over responsibility for designing much needed extensions to the hospital's buildings. Their plans were approved in 1916 and building commenced. In June 1917 a new admin-istration building and ward pavilions were opened. An impressive addition to the hospital, the new Administration Building, has been described in archi-tectural terms as:

> [a] two-level austere brick building, stylistically deriving partly from the earlier Edwardian period but also reflecting some of the Bungalow era. The Marseilles-pattern tiles were used, but in a less fanciful roof shape with a Dutch-hip as the only embellishment. The plan was a symmetrically-arranged series of bays; the central recessed bay of each faced being gabled and capped with stucco.[20]

Other improvements at this time included a large extension of the original nurses' home (later known as Yarra House), which transformed it into a three-level verandahed building.

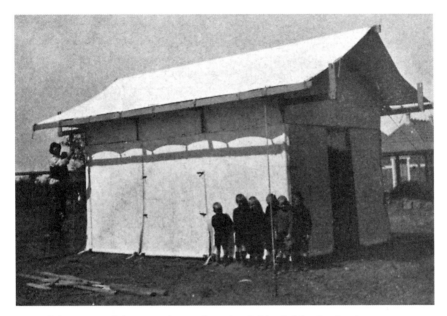

One of the tents used during epidemics (from the Golden Jubilee Brochure).

Due to community concerns about aspects of the hospital's care and administrative practices,[21] in 1912 a public inquiry was held into the affairs of the hospital. This inquiry led to an Act of Parliament in 1914. The report gives an almost Dickensian picture of aspects of the hospital's management and it is clear that in its first years of operation there were many defects—some of them extremely serious—in the running of the hospital. The report, published on 7 March 1913, was entitled *Queen's Memorial Infectious Diseases Hospital. Report of the Board of Inquiry on the Administration and General Management of, and More Particularly into the Statements Recently Made in Parliament in Connexion with the Institution; Together with an Appendix.* (No. 12, 41420). Vivian Tanner, MP was appointed to inquire into serious allegations against the hospital. Describing the activities of his one-man Board, Tanner stated: 'The inquiry was open to the public. There have been 44 sittings for the purpose of taking evidence; 156 witnesses have been examined on oath, and a transcript of their evidence is forwarded herewith. One hundred and seventy-six exhibits were put in during the course of the inquiry'. The report, the result of a thorough and broad-ranging investigation, presents a richly detailed description of aspects of the hospital's early years—years for which there is a paucity of records—and as such is worth quoting at length.

The first meeting for the hearing of evidence took place on 8 October. W. A. Sanderson appeared for the public, H. S. Cole for the secretary of the hospital, H. Crosbie, and later E. J. Corr, appeared on behalf of the committee of management. Twenty-one charges were formulated, which included:

Body of patient Samuel Waters allowed to remain in Mortuary ten days. No proper steps taken to notify relatives of death.
This charge has been conclusively proved.

The primary cause—wrong information being conveyed to the relatives of this patient—is attributable to the absence of proper particulars being placed at the disposal of the lodge porters for dissemination.

To some extent the lodge porter who gave the information that Waters was 'still improving,' when, as a matter of fact, death had actually taken place, and receiving the interrogation, 'What, is he not dead?' is blamable. Such an interrogation should have conveyed to any ordinary mind the fact that some doubt existed as to the true position of affairs, and suggested the making of further inquiry at the proper quarter . . . The fact that the body remained in the mortuary for a period of ten (10) days cannot be too severely commented upon, and reveals a state of gross mismanagement and neglect on the part of those in authority that should not have occurred in any institution.

It is within the knowledge of the secretary—the chief executive officer—that the body was in the mortuary for a period of eight (8) days yet no action was taken by him until the eighth day to further communicate with the relatives.

A similar mistake occurred in June 1911, following the admission of a patient named Matthew O'Brien. His parents were told that his condition was 'just the same', although he had actually died some hours before. As a result, the Committee of Management took steps to ensure the provision of a mortuary attendant, and a mortuary record book. A related charge was found to be proved:

No information given by post as to condition of patients. Insufficient information given by telephone and orally.
This charge is proved.

Less dissatisfaction would have arisen if, at stated intervals, parents or guardians had been supplied with brief reports by post as to the progress or otherwise of patients.

Limited information is always supplied over the telephone or upon personal inquiry at the lodge.

A number of charges of varying degrees of seriousness related to clothing, hygiene and care of patients, particular children:

Children sent to Hospital with clean heads and return home vermin infected.
This charge has been proved.

Children permitted to run about the Hospital grounds imperfectly clad and barefooted, and no action taken by the Medical Superintendent when his attention was drawn thereto.
This charge has been proved.

Girl given a man's coloured shirt for a night shirt.
This charge has been proved.

No clothing allowed to be taken to Hospital with patients from their homes, except in certain cases, when the children were taken to the institution in a night dress or shirt.
This is a medical question as to a better course to pursue. Provided proper and sufficient covering is supplied from the ambulance there should be no reason for complaint.

Patients' clothing taken to Hospital destroyed.
In one instance it has been proved that a pair of boots was destroyed during the process of fumigation, but the owner was reimbursed for the loss.

Clothing sent to convalescent patients not given to them to wear—mislaid by hospital authorities.
This charge has been proved.

Girl placed in bed with Chinese boy.
I find that in one instance a European girl was placed in bed with a half-caste Chinese boy. It may, however, be pointed out that the ages of these two children —one a European girl and the other a half-caste Chinese boy—were five and a half years and four respectively. Both were at the time very sick. Further, they were only placed in the same bed—one at each end—temporarily owing to a shortage of accommodation during an epidemic.

Children on point of death refused admission on account of the Hospital authorities not receiving a guarantee from the Municipal Councils concerned for payment of maintenance fees.
There is no evidence to support this charge.

In the year 1907 there is evidence of the refusal by the medical superinten- dent of the admission of two intending patients, but it has not been shown that they were 'on the point of death,' or that the refusals were on the grounds of the guarantees for payment not being forthcoming from the municipalities in which they resided.

Employes' [sic] clothes sent out of the hospital to be washed without first being fumigated.
This allegation has been proved.

I am of the opinion that some rule should have been framed prohibiting this course, and that provision should have been made for the washing, &c., of employes' clothes in the institution.

Bedding taken from fumigator to wards without being properly dried—children being placed in wet beds.
Bedding in some instances was not properly dried before being removed from the fumigator room, but I am satisfied from the evidence before me that such bedding was not used until thoroughly dried elsewhere.

Bedding generally in a dirty condition—straw mattresses rotten.
These allegations have been proved.

The bedding and bedclothes were only discoloured by the constant use of disinfectants and the process of fumigation. I am not satisfied from the evidence adduced that the straw mattresses were rotten, but I am of the opinion that the ticks should be refilled with fresh straw after use by each patient.

Male employees and nurses leaving Hospital grounds without changing their clothes.
So far as the male employees are concerned there is ample evidence that they repeatedly left the hospital grounds wearing the same apparel as clothed in whilst handling infected matter, and without having taken any precautions for disinfection. So far as the nurses are concerned it has not been proved that they acted similarly.

Insufficient precautions adopted by nurses to escape infection.
The evidence did not support this allegation. Reasonable precautions appear to have been taken by nurses to escape infection; notwithstanding which, a *great number* of them have contracted septic fingers. Certain medical authorities recommend the use of rubber gloves by nurses when handling septic patients.

Incinerator attendant having meals, milking cows, driving ambulance, and carrying patients without changing clothes.
This allegation has been proved.

Dead bodies carried from the wards on shoulders of attendants past children playing in grounds.
This allegation has been proved.
    Little or no precautions appear to have been taken to remove convalescent patients from the grounds whilst bodies were being conveyed to the mortuary.

Abnormal use of brandy.
This is a medical matter, and one which may well be left to the Medical Superintendent.
    In the opinion of the present Acting Medical Superintendent the use of the stimulant is an important factor in the treatment of diphtheria and scarlet fever, and his evidence goes to show that the brandy was only used medicinally.

Number of oil drums taken from Hospital grounds.
This allegation has been proved.
    Oil drums, also chaff bags, were on two occasions removed from the institution and sold, the proceeds being properly accounted for.
    The system of permitting material to be distributed outside, through the medium of trade, is most pernicious and may lead to wholesale spread of disease.

Fresh coke being tipped into pits without pits being cleaned.
This allegation has been proved.
    The pits have, however, been tested from time to time by the medical superintendent, and a bacteriological examination of three samples of water taken therefrom made by my direction for the purposes of this inquiry, failed to reveal the presence of any really deleterious matter.

Allowing cows to eat hospital refuse, &c., and using their milk for cooking purposes.
This allegation has been proved.

The practice of permitting milch cows to graze on the grounds of an infectious diseases hospital is, in my opinion, most undesirable. The letting of the hospital grounds for the grazing of sheep, as has been done, is also objectionable.

Allowing rubbish, &c., to collect about different parts of the ground.
This allegation has been proved.

Stagnant water was also permitted to remain in a drain at the rear of the stable but the drainage system now appears to be in a satisfactory condition.

Allowing iron bedsteads to remain in paddocks unprotected.
I find that this is so, but they are old and practically worthless.

Having insufficient and out-of-date laundry appliances.
This allegation has been proved.

Allowing fence to get out of repair.
On several occasions the fence at one point—across an unused quarry hole—was in a broken condition . . . Repairs were, from time to time, made as occasion arose.

Allowing stables to become dirty.
On the whole, it would appear that the stables were kept in a fairly clean condition. On specific occasions, owing to the pressure of work they were somewhat neglected for short periods.

Dissection of bodies without parents' permission.
Every phase in connexion with this matter has been most minutely inquired into and a mass of evidence taken. After a careful review thereof I am not satisfied that the allegation is proved; but taking into consideration all the circumstances surrounding the case, I am of the opinion that something more than intubation was practised on one particular body, probably tracheotomy.

It appears that a system exists at this institution of Junior medical officers appointed thereto practising intubation on bodies of patients with the knowledge of the Medical Superintendent, as tuition in this process forms no part of the medical course.

The great majority of cases treated in this institution are diphtheritic; it therefore becomes essential that medical officers appointed thereto shall at once acquaint themselves with this process. Whether their operations (other than those legally authorised) cease there, no definite evidence was forthcoming.

Any unauthorised interference with bodies in a public institution is, to my mind, objectionable.

There were a number of complaints about the secretary, most of which seem to have some basis, and also some charges about management in general:

Inebriety of secretary on or about the 29th July, 1912.
This charge has not been proved. Whilst there is evidence that this officer partook of intoxicants on the 29th of July, 1912, it has been shown that drink

was only taken at such times, and in such moderate quantities, as to at no time incapacitate him, or interfere with the performance of his duties.

Secretary obtaining receipts for wages from certain employees for amounts greater than they actually received.
This implies a charge of larceny ... the amounts short paid were properly accounted for by the secretary, whom I completely exonerate from the implied charge.
   His methods of book-keeping were, however, faulty.

Secretary seems to control the Hospital and took no notice of complaints made to him by employes [sic].
This charge has been proved.

Secretary and matron continually away from the hospital.
I find that their duties necessitated their being frequently away on business connected with the institution.

No Annual Report of secretary for some years.
This allegation has been proved, and is in breach of Rule No. 18 of the Hospital Rules and By-Laws for the guidance of the secretary. [See Queen's Memorial Hospital, first *Annual Report*, August 1915, for 16 October 1914 to 30 June 1915.]

Rules not consolidated.
This allegation has been proved.
   The rules of the institution have from time to time been amended or augmented by the committee, but no proper steps appear to have been taken to prominently bring them under the notice of the officials to whom they related. The rules relating to said officials, or groups of officials, are issued in separate form. In my opinion they should be issued in consolidated form, a copy of which should be posted up in a prominent place in the institution.
   The necessity of this was made manifest by the fact that a number of witnesses (employees) pleaded ignorance of certain rules.

No interest taken by committee in the management of the Hospital.
A perusal of the minute books show that there was a fair average attendance of members at committee meetings, but oral evidence has been given that the attendance of many of them was purely nominal and that some members merely signed the attendance book and retired shortly afterwards, taking little or no part in the deliberations of the committee. This oral evidence has not been rebutted. The committee appears to have followed the usual practice of all large committees, and delegated certain powers to a sub- or house-committee, and I am satisfied that the sub- or house-committee has not, generally, shown a lack of interest in the conduct or management of the institution.

Financial considerations, as might be expected, featured in several charges:

> *Port Melbourne Council had to sign a declaration that they would be responsible for the payment of maintenance fees for each patient admitted from within their Municipal District.*

This charge has been proved.

It is revealed by the minute books of the committee of management that the secretary, under instructions, had, from time to time, notified various municipal authorities that intending patients would not be admitted unless the necessary guarantee for the payment of maintenance fees was forthcoming but patients are not now refused admission under any circumstances when brought to the hospital.

> *Patients being charged two rates.*

This charge has been proved.

It appears from the evidence that non-contributing councils, *i.e.*, councils not contributing towards the upkeep of the institution under the provisions of the section 153 of the *Health Act* 1890, No. 1098, are charged at the rate of 7s. 6d. per patient per day, for patients from within the boundaries of their municipal districts, and the payments by the contributing councils, based in proportion to the annual assessments of the property within their areas, work out at from 3s. 9d. to 6s. 9d. per patient per day, the last-mentioned amount being now seldom reached.

I am of the opinion that the charge of 7s. 6d. per patient per day is excessive, inasmuch as it has been shown that the present cost per bed at this institution is approximately only £52 per annum.

General safety was a concern. Charges included:

> *Boiler not having been inspected for seven years, and no indication thereon as to what pressure it would stand.*

The institution is in the Shire of Heidelberg, and as the provisions of the Boilers Inspection Act do not apply to shires, there is no legal obligation to have the boiler inspected; but in view of the close proximity of the boiler-house to the laundry and kitchen, where a number of hands are employed, some inspection of the boiler should, in my opinion, have been made periodically as to its state, and a notice attached thereto showing what pressure it would, with safety, stand.

> *Insufficient precautions against fire.*

From a personal inspection of the fire appliances and a practical test of the fire hoses, from evidence given, and from the enclosed report and oral evidence of the Chief Officer of the Metropolitan Fire Brigade, I find that the precautions taken for the prevention of, and for dealing with an outbreak of, fire, are inadequate in the extreme, and the appliances practically useless and unserviceable. In an institution where there are a number of helpless patients housed, the fire appliances should, in my opinion, be up-to-date and regularly inspected, and fire drill regularly carried out by certain members of the staff.

The permitting of the long growth of grass in the immediate vicinity of some of the tent wards may lead to dire consequences, as in the summer time it becomes dry and is easily ignited. [See also Tanner Report, p. 13, Appendix prepared by H. B. Lee, Metropolitan Fire Brigade].

Allowing boiler fire to be kept going all night, whilst one Falkingham was engineer, with no one in attendance.
This allegation has been proved.

Not having sufficient male staff, necessitating those employed working long hours.
This allegation has been proved.

The staff has now been increased.

There was justifiable concern about the hospital ambulance service:

Ambulance service not sufficient for the needs of a city like Melbourne.
It is obvious that the ambulance service, which consists of two one-horse vehicles—one for diphtheria and the other for scarlet fever patients—(one being on loan from the Health Department), is not sufficient for Melbourne and suburbs, in consequence of which intending patients have frequently been kept from four to five hours in the ambulance, owing to the number of patients to be collected and the long distances to be traversed—the lives of such persons being thereby endangered.

The equipment of the vehicles is also inadequate, there being no provision for either drinking water or stimulants; neither have proper means been taken to thoroughly disinfect the vehicles after each trip.

In many cases probationary or inexperienced nurses have been sent out on ambulance duty, which is a further menace to the lives of intending patients. The fact that on one occasion the ambulance had to call at the Alfred Hospital for the purpose of having anti-toxin injected into a patient shows the necessity of having experienced nurses for this duty.

A practice very much to be condemned is followed by nurses and drivers on ambulance duty, *i.e.*, making use of public and hotel telephones, after being in infected and handling infected persons, to convey messages to, or receive instructions from, the hospital authorities. This practice is, to my mind, most dangerous as it has been proved that no precautionary measures are taken beforehand.

The report commented on the lack of an observation ward, poor facilities for visitors and for preliminary examination of patients, and the inadequate kitchen and laundry:

In addition to the charges and allegations herein dealt with, I find that this institution is without an 'Observation' ward. The necessity for such a ward is obvious, and has constantly been emphasised by various Medical Superintendents, including the present Acting Medical Superintendent.

There is evidence that persons have been admitted, ostensibly suffering from [diphtheria] or scarlet fever and after having been placed in the wards where those diseases are treated, it has been ascertained on further examination that they were suffering from some complaint other than diphtheria or scarlet fever.

It appears from the minute-books of the hospital that the committee of management has, for some years, been seized by the importance of having such a ward, but strange to say, they have not taken any decisive action for the erection of the same.

It has been sworn that, for the want of funds, this ward was not established. By an examination of the records I find that this is not borne out.

The accommodation provided for [those] visiting convalescent patients and for the patients themselves, on visiting days is most crude and unsatisfactory, and causes a great amount of friction and complaint by visiting relatives. The system in existence consists of two enclosures, 66 feet apart, without any shelter from the elements.

The permanent head of the Health Department, in a report on this institution dated 20th September, 1910, recommended the following, in which I concur:–

> I would recommend that a room be provided, for visits to convalescent patients at the boundary fence. The wall of separation could be furnished with a window and a grille. The patient would be in one room and the visitor in another, and though they could see and converse with, they cannot touch each other—the access to patients' room being quite separate and distinct from that to the visitors' room. The visitor's room could also be made an inquiry depot for visitors desiring to make personal inquiry as to the welfare of patients, or to inspect the 'State of Health' book, at a stated hour every day.

This recommendation was not, however, followed, the enclosures referred to being substituted. . . . The kitchen and laundry at this institution are totally inadequate, and the appliances, fittings, &c., are obsolete . . . No proper place for the preliminary examination of patients and the obtaining of particulars regarding them upon their arrival at the hospital are provided: the former is usually carried out in the ambulance and the particulars are obtained on the verandah of the Receiving House (which is also used as a Discharging House) when attending at the request of the authorities for the purpose of removing convalescent patients.

Other comments included:

> It frequently happens that intending patients are conveyed to the hospital in cabs, and these vehicles are permitted to depart after undergoing what appears to me to be an inefficient process of disinfection, consequently the danger of the wholesale spreading of infection by these public vehicles is great . . .
>
> The incinerator used for the destruction of excreta, &c., from the wards and lavatories, and other places is inefficient, and is in an unsuitable position; I also find that the manner in which the matter for destruction is conveyed thereto is most objectionable.

The installing of an up-to-date incinerator has engaged the attention of the hospital authorities on more than one occasion, but action to procure one has been deferred.

A matter which is frequently voiced in no mild language by parents and relatives is the long detention of some patients, apparently cured, in the hospital. I am, however, of the opinion that there is no cause for complaint in this direction. Some patients who, after a period of treatment appear to be in a perfect state of health, are germ carriers, and their liberation would be a menace to the public generally. No patient is detained in the institution longer than is absolutely necessary ...

In view of the average number of patients treated at this hospital I am of the opinion that the permanent ward accommodation is altogether inadequate, and the use of 'tents,' originally erected as temporary expedients, are, and have been for some time, in constant use, and appear to be regarded as 'permanent accommodation.'

The report was concerned with the staffing situation. A large proportion of the nurses employed at the hospital were probationers and even more were trainees; there were very few qualified nurses employed. The hospital also had difficulty obtaining wardsmaids, and nurses were forced to undertake extra work 'to the detriment of their professional duties.' The fairly rapid turnover of medical superintendents and assistant medical officers was also noted.

The segregation of convalescent patients was described as 'woefully lax'. Diphtheria and scarlet fever wards were within a few yards of one another, without even a dividing fence. It was also mentioned that convalescent patients absconded due to lack of supervision. The report concluded:

I may add that I am satisfied that the patients at this hospital are generally well treated, and in my opinion it speaks well for the institution that during the last three years, with the daily average of patients of 120, 159, and 165, the percentage of deaths from all diseases treated shows 3.84, 3.9, and 5.04 respectively ...

As will be seen from the report, the evidence of 156 witnesses covered 2,100 odd pages of foolscap. The exhibits were also numerous ...

An appendix to the report, 'By an Officer of the Brigade on Infectious Diseases Hospital, Fairfield,' was prepared by H. B. Lee of the Metropolitan Fire Brigade:

I have the honour to report having visited the Infectious Diseases Hospital Fairfield. This hospital consists of a number of brick and wooden single-story buildings.

The wooden buildings are of such a construction that they would be destroyed very quickly in the event of an outbreak of fire. The doors in the building should be made wide enough to permit of a bed with the patient in it being removed at a moments notice. In some of the wooden buildings this could not be done . . . In the event of one of the wooden buildings becoming well alight, no adequate means are provided for the extinction of the fire.

There is a very obsolete incinerator in a wooden shed in dangerous proximity to a wooden stable and hay-loft. This I consider should be immediately removed and replaced by an effective destructor placed in an isolated position.

In the laundry . . . At present it is dangerous.

The buildings are all lighted with gas, but during certain hours kerosene lamps are used about the place, and, as I understand it would not involve much expense but in fact would be an economy, I would recommend that electric lighting apparatus be installed and the buildings and grounds lighted by electricity, thus dispensing with the kerosene lamps for the grounds and the danger of lighted matches from the gas.

While lamps are used at the hospital I would recommend the lamp room or such place in the laundry which is used in this capacity be removed and some shed remote from the hospital buildings be used for this purpose . . .

We are fortunate to have such a detailed report. Some of the evidence presented does not reflect well on the hospital and its staff. But it is worth noting that the hospital had been fully operational for only eight years when the investigation took place and was still finding its feet as a new hospital designed to tackle difficult medical problems in a field where few people had much experience or skill. The report concentrates—as it was meant to do—on the deficiencies and failings of the hospital and thus tends to ignore the more positive aspects of its health care standards and administration. Having said this, there can be no doubt that some serious problems existed and that the hospital had—due to inexperience—fallen into a good many inefficient and dangerous practices.

The report provided a much needed opportunity to make a fresh start and, importantly, led to an improvement in the hospital's financial position. One of the first positive developments emanating from the Tanner Inquiry was the setting up of a new Finance Sub-committee. The speed with which the hospital pursued this initiative reflected the urgency of its financial situation. At the first meeting held in the Melbourne Town Hall on 20 October 1913, chaired by Cr Allard, the sub-committee examined the hospital ledger and 'instructed' the secretary of the hospital to send to each council that owed the hospital money a letter requesting that it settle its account as soon as possible.[22] At its next meeting on 5 November the sub-committee, in fiery Guy Fawkes Day mood, rejected the softly, softly approach to the hospital's debtors favoured by the hospital's honorary solicitor and the secretary and insisted that accounts be immediately rendered to councils that owed the hospital money. It was, however, prepared to 'effect a compromise' with respect to the Shire of Upper Yarra, which was indebted to the tune of £245 7s 6d and had asked if it could negotiate a reduced payment. There was 'considerable discussion' at this meeting regarding the hospital's financial position and it would appear that the sub-committee was unhappy about lack of information regarding the hospital's finances. The secretary asked that a further meeting be held at which he would present a 'proper Financial Statement'.

At this meeting, on 10 November 1913, the financial report presented by the secretary showed that the hospital was owed a small fortune in unpaid accounts. Contributing councils owed almost half of the total debt: Melbourne, £570 10s 9d; Malvern, £61 7s 10d, Brunswick, £59; Williamstown, £25 10s 5d; and Coburg, £19 12s—a total of £736 1s 4d. Non-contributing councils had been allowed to build up even larger debts: Brighton, £353 5s; Caulfield, £281 17s 6d; Camberwell, £258 14s; Essendon, £298 7s 6d; Upper Yarra Shire, £100. Shipping companies (on account of emigrants) owed £210. The secretary informed the sub-committee that a £500 overdraft appeared in the accounts as an estimated receipt; this 'was not a strictly correct entry' and that the overdraft would be completely expended in the 'current quarter'. In attempting to tidy up a financial situation which had been allowed to slide more or less out of control prior to the Tanner Inquiry, the sub-committee decided to cut its losses and write off all outstanding accounts that had been 'repudiated by Councils'. This sub-committee was to play an important role in providing sound and sensible financial leadership for the hospital in the years ahead—this type of financial scrutiny and leadership had been somewhat lacking in the hospital since its opening in 1904.

The Tanner Report, which was presented to the Premier of Victoria on 7 March 1913, led to the passing of the *Queen's Memorial Infectious Diseases Hospital Act* in 1914. This Act provided for a Board of Management consisting of six government and six municipal representatives, the whole of the metropolitan councils being brought under the Act. The first meeting of the new Board took place on 16 October 1914 at the offices of the Department of Health. The hospital's first annual report published in August 1915, provided a detailed description of the structure of the new Board:

> The Board consists of twelve members, six appointed by the Governor-in Council, one elected by the Council of the City of Melbourne, and one elected by each of the five groups of municipalities mentioned in the first Schedule of the Act. The members were Mrs. J. J. Brenan, Mrs. Hay, Dr F. Miller Johnson, Dr A. Jeffreys Wood, Councillor J. H. Gardiner, and Councillor J. H. Stone, representing the government; Alderman William Strong, elected by the City of Melbourne; Councillors E. Coulson, W. E. Cash, Rupert de C. Wilks, Thomas Smith and B. J. Ferdinando, elected by the Groups A, B, C, D, and E, respectively. The Municipalities mentioned are as follow:–

Group A:The Municipalities of Collingwood, Fitzroy, Richmond, Heidelberg.
Group B:The Municipalities of Williamstown, Footscray, Braybrook, Essendon, Coburg, Brunswick, Preston, Northcote.
Group C: The Municipalities of Malvern, Hawthorn, Kew, Camberwell, Nunawading, Dandenong.
Group D:The Municipalities of Port Melbourne, South Melbourne, St. Kilda, Brighton.
Group E:The Municipalities of Prahran, Caulfield, Moorabbin, Oakleigh.
Upper Yarra was added to Group C on 1st January 1915, and Epping to Group A on 1st April, 1915.
Alderman Strong was unanimously elected Chair of the Board for the first term.

Sub-Committees
Mrs. Brenan, Dr Johnson, Councillors Cash, Coulson, Gardiner and Stone were elected to form a House Committee.

Mrs Hay, Dr Wood, Councillors Cash, Ferdinando, Smith and Wilks, were elected to form a Finance Committee, Cr. Cash being appointed Chair. Mrs Hay retired in November, 1914, Mrs. A. Holdaway being appointed to fill the vacancy. Dr F. Miller Johnson, having enlisted as a medical officer with the Australian Expeditionary Forces, resigned in March 1915, and Dr James Amess was appointed in his place. The Board have to record, with sincere regret, the death of the Chair (Alderman William Strong), which occurred on 25th April 1915. Alderman Strong was practically the founder of the Hospital, having initiated the public subscription for a memorial of the late Queen Victoria, it being subsequently decided that the amount subscribed (about £10,000) should be expended in the erection of the Infectious Diseases Hospital. He was also Chair of the Committee of Management almost from the inception until that Committee gave way to the present Board of Management. The Board takes this opportunity of expressing its appreciation of the valuable services rendered to the Hospital by the late Alderman. As a memorial an enlarged photograph has been obtained and placed in the Administration Block at the Hospital. The vacant position of Chair of the Board was filled by the election of Councillor Thomas Smith. Councillor William Andrews was elected by the City of Melbourne as representative in place of Alderman Strong.

Under the provisions of the Act, the total expenditure is contributed to the Board in equal proportions by (a) the Contributing Municipalities, and (b) the Treasurer of Victoria. 30 Ann. Rep, 1915.

The publication of this first—and very belated—annual report coincided with the appointment of A. A. Marsden as secretary of the hospital, a post he held for twenty-four years. The year 1915 also saw the passing of the *Health Act*, a consolidation Act (customary every twenty-five years). This Act incorporated some of the recommendations of an advisory committee on infectious disease set up following an epidemic of cerebro-spinal meningitis.

Cerebro-spinal meningitis (epidemic meningitis, cerebro-spinal fever, spinal meningitis, meningococcus meningitis and spotted or petechial fever) was first recognised as a specific disease in Geneva in 1805. The organism responsible was identified in 1807, when Anton Weichselbaum isolated the meningococcus and named it *Diplococcus intracellularis meningitides*, though the name was later changed to *Neisseria meningitidis*. From 1837 to 1850 there were a number of epidemics throughout Europe, and the disease was rampant in military camps during both world wars. There were only sporadic cases in Australia in the nineteenth century, but in 1915 there was an Australia-wide epidemic, starting in Victoria and South Australia, that continued till 1918. It is generally a childhood infection with babies most at risk, however outbreaks occur in crowded conditions such as military barracks. Fever, pallor, headache, vomiting and lethargy are characteristic symptoms. A rash and neck stiffness may develop. The disease responds to antibiotics. Cerebrospinal meningitis occurs sporadically world wide, with occasional epidemics.

The first annual report provides an interesting account of the functioning of the hospital and how it was coping with the demands made upon it and the particular problems caused by Australia's involvement in World War I:

> In the following Statement of Receipts and Expenditure it will be observed that the Expenditure for the six months ended 30th June, 1915, exceeded the Estimates as approved. This excess was caused partly by the increased prices of commodities and partly by the fact that the daily average of patients was estimated on the figures for the previous year, viz., 125, the actual daily average being 155, an increase of nearly 25 per cent. A corresponding increase in the number of Nurses was necessary.

> *Medical Staff*
> During the latter half of the term under review, owing to the existing conditions [World War I], the Board was unable to maintain the Medical Staff of the Hospital at its proper strength. The two Assistant Medical Officers were, in February, accepted for active service by the Imperial government, and it was not until three months later that the position of Senior Assistant was filled by the appointment of Dr Rachel Champion.
> The position of Second Assistant is still vacant.
> The Board is indebted to the Honourable the Minister for Education for permitting Dr Harvey Sutton to take up the position of Resident Super-

intendent during the illness of Dr Scholes in April, and to Dr Scholes for carrying on the work of the hospital without assistance, and immediately after his illness for several weeks.

Medical Superintendent's Report

... Report on the work done in the Hospital during the nine-months ended 30th June, 1915 ... The total number of days' stay in Hospital was 39,379, and the daily average of patients 144.2. The minimum number of patients in the Hospital was 101, on November 27th, and the maximum number 213, on April 8th. These wide variations, together with the fact that it is impossible to accurately foretell the number of patients requiring accommodation, render the working of the Hospital very difficult, particularly in regard to staffing and supplies. The wards have been at times very crowded ...

The medical superintendent reported on the statistics for the major diseases treated. Of the 1351 patients treated for diphtheria, 1243 were admitted, 1140 discharged and 63 died, while 148 remained in hospital on 30 June 1915. The case mortality was 5.15 per cent, however eleven deaths occurred within twenty-four hours of admission—if these were discounted, the percentage mortality was reduced to 4.29. He commented:

During the last six years a change in type of diphtheria has taken place in Melbourne, and in my experience diphtheria is a much more serious disease than it was six years ago. Laryngeal diphtheria is very much less frequent, due largely no doubt to the practice of sending patients for treatment at an earlier stage of the disease. But to counterbalance this, the disease has taken on a more severe form, and a very large proportion of the cases now admitted are of a malignant form, attacking chiefly children from four to fifteen years of age; that is, of school age. Certain schools have been particularly affected. In many of these cases treatment is quite ineffectual, though applied at an early stage of the disease.

The incidence of scarlet fever was lower than diphtheria, and the mortality also was lower. Of the 135 patients treated from 1 July to 30 June, two died—however both the fatal cases were complicated with other diseases on admission. Measles also had a low incidence and mortality compared with diphtheria. Ninety-four patients were treated, and there were no deaths—but as most of the patients were adults, a high mortality was not expected. Four other deaths occurred—from bronchopneumonia, cerebellar haemorrhage, abdominal tuberculosis, and septic pharyngitis. The death from bronchopneumonia occurred five hours after admission, as did that from abdominal tuberculosis.

In regard to facilities and accommodation, the report commented:

During the year patients suffering from measles were housed in military tents, and later another tent was borrowed from the Health Department. These have now been replaced by more suitable structures with floors, and nurses' duty rooms and annexes are now approaching completion. I still consider that this provision is highly unsatisfactory, and welcome the decision of the Board that they are to be regarded merely as temporary structures. A few improvements have been effected in connection with the scarlet fever buildings, but they still remain quite unfit for the purposes to which they are being put.

Two motor ambulances were obtained during the year. This innovation has facilitated the quick removal of patients to a certain extent, but owing to the greatly increased area which the Board is now expected to serve, this advantage has been largely discounted. Delays still constantly occur, and an examination of the facts will show that two ambulances are insufficient for the work to be done.

A special committee, appointed to consider the terms of training, and staffing details recommended that the term for probationer nurses be altered from six to twelve months, that trained nurses be altered from six to twelve months, that trained nurses attending for their infectious diseases course be required to do four months, instead of three, and that the term for nurses who were pupils at other hospitals be altered from three to six months. The recommendation was also made that staff should include four sisters and six staff nurses for the proper supervision of the wards and nurse training. These recommendations were adopted by the Board.

A sub-committee was appointed to consider and report on a schedule of necessary works prepared by the Medical Superintendent. It recommended that a ward for 40 scarlet fever patients, a ward for 24 measles patients, a nurses' home with accommodation for 60 nurses, a larger discharging block, with store-room for linen etc. and patients' clothes, a 'shelter house' for visitors and patients visited be 'proceeded with as soon as possible'. The sewering of the hospital, the installation of electric light and a power plant for the laundry, and the extension or rebuilding of the kitchen were also high priorities. The next step was to obtain funding, and so a deputation waited upon the Minister of Health with this request:

> that the Board be granted power to borrow for Capital Expenditure upon the same basis as the Metropolitan Asylums Board (London) which controls certain Fever Hospitals. The Minister recognised the necessity of the work, and stated that while the government proportion of the total expenditure (approximately £25,000) could be paid when required, he would submit the question of giving the Board borrowing powers to the Cabinet, provided the consent of the Municipalities interested were obtained. That content is now being sought, and the Board hopes, during the current year, to obtain the necessary power and to be able to carry out the most urgent of the items in the Schedule. Unless borrowing power be obtained for the necessary capital expenditure, any expenditure so incurred would have to be added to the annual assessments, which would be very embarrassing to the municipalities . . . Thos. J. Smith. Chair.[23]

An isolation and observation block, containing twelve separate wards of varying sizes was being constructed (at a cost of £2780). The Board anticipated a further expenditure (of approximately £500) for necessary for furnishing, medical and surgical equipment and connection with water and hot-water services and covered pathways. Two large floored tents were erected as temporary provision for cases of measles. A lawn was made for the convalescent patients in Ward 5, 'it having been proved', as the Board commented, 'that these lawns save work for the Nursing Staff, in that the children can play in the open air without getting dirty'. Other expenses included an extension of 200 feet to the water main, as a precaution against fire in the scarlet fever wards, fencing for verandahs, alteration of the coach house to accommodate two ambulance cars, and planting shelter trees.

Clearly the first years of the hospital's operations were most difficult and demanding ones. To say that it experienced some teething problems would be to understate the magnitude of the difficulties. It is also clear that the hospital did not, in these early years, cope well with the demands placed upon it and that mistakes, both minor and major, were made. Importantly, however, the problems—not all of which were of the hospital's own making—were publicly aired, and radical and effective interventions were made which set the hospital upon a much firmer footing and allowed it to begin to lay the solid foundations upon which it could start to build an excellent medical facility.

Queen's Memorial Infectious Diseases Hospital
1919–1947

> We have been slow to understand that we live in a new biocultural era. For decades we cherished the myth that infectious diseases were fading forever. This was a posture born of inherited optimism. The nineteenth century generated an almost religious faith in social, scientific and technological progress. Such optimism enabled people to call the slaughter of 1914–1918 a war to end all wars. The two great global epidemics of that era, typhus and type A influenza, each killed 20 million people or more, dwarfing the toll of combat, without blunting faith in medical progress.
>
> Arno Karlen, *Plague's Progress*, p. 3.

A N INFLUENZA EPIDEMIC popularly known as 'Spanish flu' killed at least 20 million people from the spring of 1918 till 1919 in Europe, the United States and India. The flu was labelled Spanish flu because Alfonso XIII of Spain was among its first victims—and a right royal contagion it was to turn out to be. The influenza was first noted in Europe in May 1918, when the war was still in progress. Members of the AIF on active service on the Western Front were the first Australian victims, with 209 infected soldiers dying in British military hospitals. Troop ships returning to Australia at the cessation of hostilities were subject to major outbreaks of the virus. The first of these infected ships arrived in Australia in October 1918, and they were placed under quarantine restrictions which banned disembarkation until seven days after the last reported case of influenza on the vessel. That men, many of whom had survived the worst of the fighting on Gallipoli and the Western Front, should have died when their fighting days were over and they were returning home is an irony almost beyond tragedy.

Despite precautions, the influenza pandemic spread to Victoria, almost certainly via men from the 1st AIF being repatriated to Australia. Some 3530 people died from this influenza in 1919 and a further 326 deaths were recorded from broncho-pneumonia and pneumonia, many of which were directly linked to the influenza virus. The pressure on medical resources was so severe that doctors returning to Australia from military service overseas were asked to begin treating patients as soon as they disembarked. The cavernous Exhibition Buildings (where the Victorian Parliament sat, because the federal Parliament was using the state parliament buildings pending the construction of the federal parliament in the new capital, Canberra) became an emergency hospital.[1] In Fitzroy, a poor inner-suburb of Melbourne, for example, 2559 serious cases of the influenza were reported (mild cases were not reported) and over 100 deaths were recorded as being directly linked to the influenza outbreak. In response to delays in getting influenza victims admitted to hospital, Fitzroy Council, with the assistance of local residents, converted Bell Street School into 'a perfect little hospital'.[2] Many other schools and public buildings throughout Victoria and the nation as a whole were used as emergency hospital accommodation.

The influenza outbreak caused great alarm and fear in the community. People tried to avoid contact with others as much as possible, and many wore masks whenever they had to move about in public. Social life was, of course, much affected, because public gatherings constituted health risks. Many church congregations stopped meeting in their church buildings and held all services in the open air like the Covenanters of old. While in the main the community united to face and fight the influenza scourge, there were some problems between neighbouring states and in some instances state borders were closed in an attempt to stop the infection spreading. Miners in Kalgoorlie, for example, hijacked the Trans-Continental train and held it for three months in a vain attempt to stop the influenza virus being 'imported' into Western Australia. Fortunately, despite the high level of fear, this type of overreaction was rare and the community as a whole recognised the importance of remaining calm and working together.

Queens's Memorial Hospital was, of course, deeply involved in efforts to treat influenza victims and during the course of the epidemic acted under the instructions of the Central Influenza Authority established by the government. The Victorian Minister for Public Health in November 1918 asked the Hospital Board to reserve a Ward Pavilion (which was then unoccupied) exclusively for influenza patients, as these beds might be needed if the epidemic increased. By the end of January 1919, the epidemic having worsened, this reservation was taken up. The two wards in the pavilion were opened and filled with patients almost immediately. Within a fortnight the hospital opened another ward for influenza patients, thus bringing the number of beds exclusively devoted to influenza patients to ninety. The cost, maintenance and medical and nursing staff of these wards were provided by the Public Health Department.

Influenza, a potentially lethal disease commonly known as flu, is caused by a group of myxoviruses designated types A, B and (debatably) C. Influenza B and C usually cause only mild symptoms. Influenza A, however, can cause pandemics, such as occurred in 1918–19. (It was referred to as 'Flanders Grippe' by English soldiers, 'Blitz Katarrh' by German troops, 'wrestler fever' by the Japanese, and 'Spanish Flu' or, more poetically, 'Spanish Lady' by Americans.) Flu was first recorded in Australia in 1820, and epidemics continue to occur Australia-wide with gloomy regularity. The devastating pandemic which started in Europe in 1918 reached Melbourne in January 1919 and was declared a quarantinable disease under the Commonwealth Quarantine Act.

Influenza was first described by Hippocrates in BCE 412. Symptoms may include fever, malaise, headache and myalgia. The spread of influenza can be very rapid from country to country, and is particularly dangerous because the virus can mutate quickly. A leading medical authority in Melbourne in 1890 stated 'the [flu] epidemic is propagated by letters or merchandise', but the common view at the time was that the disease was spread 'on the wings of the wind' by 'noxious breezes', and it was commonly called 'fog fever'. However, a report on influenza in New South Wales in 1891 concluded the disease is transmitted from person to person directly, by inhaling infected 'secretions of the mouth and lungs'. In the past, people have tried preventive measures such as tying cucumbers to their ankles, adding sulphur to their shoes, gargling with vinegar and water and wearing white cotton masks at all times except when eating or washing. Vaccinations have succeeded in reducing mortality and morbidity, but the influenza virus is still a formidable enemy, and is likely to take its toll for many years to come.

During the course of the epidemic the hospital admitted 1305 influenza patients, of whom 120 died, the mortality rate being 9.2 per cent. Interestingly, hospital records show that nearly all the patients admitted suffering from influenza were female. Sandland has suggested that this gender imbalance is 'probably a commentary on the fact that many of their menfolk had already had it at the war front, and that the effects of the virus on children did not induce classical symptoms, though upper respiratory tract infections, severe croup or even diarrhoeal illness could be produced'.[3]

The wards 'loaned' to the government during the epidemic were closed on 8 September 1919. The government, however, reflecting on the acute pressure the epidemic had placed on hospital resources, in December 1919 obtained the hospital Board's permission to place temporary buildings on hospital land to provide emergency accommodation in the event of a further influenza outbreak. Perhaps as a result of the influenza epidemic, in 1919 the Hospital Board, chaired by Cr W. E. Cash, decided to appoint a resident bacteriologist. This decision was an important step towards building the hospital's pro-active, research-based approach to treating and combating infectious diseases.

The Victorian Parliament passed a new *Health Act* on 6 January 1919, replacing the Board of Public Health with a seven-member Commission of Public Health. The Act consolidated all existing Health Acts and incorporated further provisions from British Health Acts. The Act has been seen as marking a notable advance in public health theory and practice in Victoria. The new legislation divided Victoria into six health areas, each of which was supervised by a district health officer—a full-time medical officer employed by the state government. The Act, moreover, designated each municipality as the local health authority, required to appoint a qualified medical practitioner as medical officer and a health inspector. In terms of infectious disease control, the Act constituted considerable progress, stressing as it did the importance of research and education. The general tenor of the Act is shown in its statement of objectives:

> [to] promote the prevention, limitation and suppression of infectious and preventable diseases; to report to the Minister upon matters affecting the public health ... to publish reports, information and advice concerning the public health and, in particular, concerning the prevention of disease and the education of the public in the preservation of health.[4]

The influenza epidemic resulted in Queen's Memorial Hospital recording an increased admission of over 1000 patients between June 1918 and June 1919. To put this in perspective, diphtheria admissions were much higher than this—they were 2612 during the same period, and in the previous three years had been similar, at 2478, 2442 and 2361.

The hospital continued to have difficulty in obtaining qualified medical officers and in 1918/19 was forced to resort once again (for the fifth year) to appointing fifth-year medical students. Following the decision made during the influenza epidemic, Dr Helen Kelsey was appointed in 1919 as a resident bacteriologist, and the Board was pleased to note that the 'laboratory equipment is now fairly complete'.

In the annual report for 1918/19, the Medical Superintendent, Dr Scholes, noted that nursing staff levels remained 'very unsatisfactory', with the result that patients were 'being refused admission, not because there is no room for them, but because there are positively no nurses to nurse them'. Scholes clearly considered that this problem was outside his power to control and simply stated 'I would ask the Board to consider the position'. It would appear from this somewhat cryptic comment that Scholes felt the Board had the capacity to make the finance available which would make the hospital more competitive in attracting nurses. In the 1919/20 annual report, Scholes analysed the hospital's staffing position:

> The resident medical staff has been kept well up to strength during the year. The nursing position, however, remained unsatisfactory throughout the year. Not only do the patients in the wards suffer on account of the shortage, but during the busy periods of the year scores of children were refused admission because the already overworked nurses could not attend to any more patients.
>
> The shortage of probationer nurses is largely due to the fact that fever hospital nursing is, and has been for many years, in some ways a blind alley. After passing through her period of training (12–18 months), passing her examination, and becoming entitled to her Infectious Diseases certificate, she is compelled to return to the beginning and go through the whole of her period of training at a general hospital. Not only is no credit given for the time spent and knowledge acquired, but she cannot be granted her Infectious certificate until she gains her General one.
>
> Negotiations are in progress with the Royal Victorian Trained Nurses' Association, and an arrangement is hoped for which will be satisfactory to all concerned.

In the 1921 annual report, Scholes was still very concerned about the staffing situation regarding nurses, although he did have some positive developments to report:

> During March and April . . . the nursing position became so acute that admission of patients was perforce curtailed, there being insufficient nurses to attend to them. The Board effected important alterations to the salary scale, and in conditions of work, with satisfactory results. I am of the opinion, however, that the position will remain difficult until such time as the nurses are given official recognition of the work done. The statements made by me [regarding the lack of a career path] in my last annual report still hold good.

Scholes was also pleased to note that the Board had approved the construction of a pavilion (two wards) for measles and whooping cough patients, and of a store for bedding, mattresses and beds, and that work on these extensions to the hospital's facilities had already started. On 28 July 1922 these were

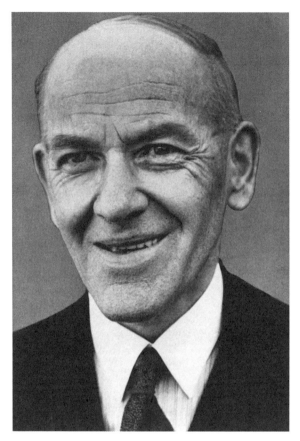

Dr F. V. Scholes, Medical Superintendent, 1910–48

opened by Matthew Baird, Minister for Public Health. But another epidemic was soon to put the hospital's limited resources to the test:

> In November 1919, a severe epidemic [of measles] arose in the northern suburbs and extended throughout Melbourne during the following months. Many thousands of cases occurred, but owing to the lack of accommodation, the patients received at Fairfield were limited practically to those with complications, and even so a considerable number of cases with broncho-pneumonia were perforce refused. Under the circumstances the mortality rate of 12.33 per cent. is considered satisfactory. Many of the deaths [46] were of constitutionally weak and starved children. Six deaths occurred within 24 hours of admission.

The measles (morbilli) epidemic 'died out in August' 1920.

Measles, also known as morbilli or rubeola, is an acute, highly infectious viral disease which is spread by airborne droplets and is most common in children. Symptoms include fever, severe catarrh and a rash. One attack of measles will confer immunity, so after an epidemic there are only sporadic outbreaks until a new generation of susceptible children appear. A Persian physician, Rhazes (Abu Becr Mohammed Ibn Zacariya Ar-Razi) wrote a book about 900CE distinguishing measles from smallpox, however in the sixteenth century it was still common for the title 'smallpoxe and mesles' to be applied to a single illness. The name is derived from 'miselli', a diminutive of 'miser', and was used by John of Gaddeseden in the fourteenth century instead of the Latin word '*morbilli*'. The disease spread from Europe, causing devastation whenever it was introduced to a previously unexposed population, and is now world wide. Measles was introduced into Victoria in 1850, brought on the ship *Persian*. An effective vaccine was discovered in 1960, and routine vaccination of babies has greatly reduced the mortality from this disease.

Victoria had a potentially very serious smallpox scare in 1921, when a fireman from a ship docked in Melbourne was taken to the Melbourne hospital, diagnosed as suffering from malaria and admitted. It soon became obvious that he had been misdiagnosed and that he was in fact suffering from smallpox. By this time he had already infected two people. A further six cases were diagnosed at Geelong, and for a short time it looked possible that Victoria was on the verge of a major smallpox epidemic. Investigations could prove no link between the infections in Melbourne and the Geelong outbreak, but it would be a remarkable coincidence if the two were unconnected—particularly as these infections have the distinction of being the last recorded smallpox cases in Victoria.

In the 1921/22 annual report, Scholes presents a wonderfully concise description of the management dilemmas created by the seasonal and wildly fluctuating demands on hospital facilities which are inherent in the role of an infectious diseases hospital:

> The year has been a quiet one on the whole. As usual, the diphtheria admissions were light during the summer months. The autumnal wave was later and much less marked than had been the case for several years, with the result that the total number of admissions for the year fell far short of expectations.

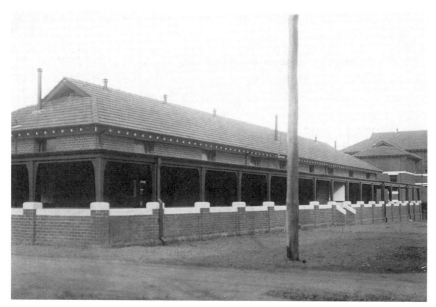

Ward 12, built in 1922 to house polio patients and photographed in 1937.

Herein lies one of the chief difficulties of fever hospital management and finance. Preparations must be made for the annual autumnal increase, and the staff brought up far beyond its summer strength. It is safe to prophesy that the period March–September will be the busiest period of the year, but no idea can be gained beforehand as to the number of admissions, or the maximum number of beds that will be required. Thus in 1921, from a minimum of 170 in January, a maximum of 600 was reached in May; while this year, starting from approximately the same minimum, the maximum reached was only 430.

There were seasonal patterns of infectious disease which enabled the hospital to make general provisions for estimated demands, but the patterns had such wide variations that even short-term plans were subject to sudden and extreme variables, and all plans for the management and finance of the hospital were of necessity contingency plans. An infectious disease hospital is subject to sudden and often extreme demands and can be transformed in a matter of days from being very much under-utilised and overstaffed to bursting at the seams and grossly understaffed.

Scholes noted two other significant events in his report on the previous year's activities. In relation to diphtheria the news was very positive:

> deaths from diphtheria were fewer than for many years, and the percentage mortality the lowest in the history of the hospital [2.2 per cent]. The mildness of the type of diphtheria has been a factor in producing this result; but another

factor should not be ignored, the increased use of the intravenous route in injecting antitoxin.

On a darker note, Scholes also stated that 'At a Conference held to consider the question of possible Plague [the infamous 'Black Death'] infection in Victoria, an agreement was reached that, in the event of space being available, patients suffering from the bubonic form of the disease would be accommodated at Fairfield.

The introductory pages to the 1922/23 annual report included an attractively bordered one paragraph description of the hospital and its work:

> The hospital is situated at Fairfield, in the Shire of Heidelberg, and is built in an area of land granted by the Crown, and containing about 22 acres. There is a further area of about 22 acres, adjoining the hospital for extensions in the future. The hospital contains 563 beds, set apart for the treatment of patients suffering from Diphtheria, Scarlet Fever, Measles, Whooping Cough, Cerebrospinal Meningitis, Infantile Paralysis and Influenza. The accommodation for patients consists of 16 large wards, and 36 small wards. A Motor Ambulance Service is maintained for the transport of patients to the hospital.

This description, with only minor changes to note the increasing size of the hospital, appeared at the front of the annual report for fifteen years. In the

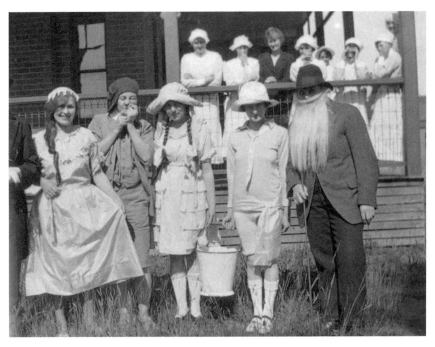

Staff dressed up for a concert party and pantomime in 1921, outside the nurses home.

Bubonic plague/Pneumonic plague is the 'Black Death' which caused the devastating pandemic of 1346–50, wiping out about half the population of Europe. It is probably the disease that slew the Philistines, mentioned in the Old Testament Book of Samuel—'they had emerods (swellings) in their secret parts'. It is caused by the bacterium *Pasteurella pestis*; it infects both rats and humans, and is transmitted by fleas. The pneumonic form does not require a flea vector but can be transmitted by droplets from person to person. Fever, buboes (swollen lymph nodes), and bleeding under the skin causing blackish blotches, are symptoms of bubonic plague, and pneumonic plague is characterised by a fulminating pneumonia. The last major outbreak in Europe occurred in 1664–65 (the Great Plague of London was part of this pandemic), and plague inexplicably decreased in Europe from this time on. Plague spread slowly in the Far East during 1894–99 and made its first appearance in Australian ports, including Melbourne, in 1900. However, there were only 12 cases reported in Victoria from 1900 to 1909, and only a few isolated cases in all Australia from 1910 onwards. A vaccine now exists and plague can usually be successfully treated with antibiotics.

1937/38 annual report, it had expanded to 720 beds in 20 large wards and 36 small wards. The list of diseases treated no longer contained meningitis or whooping cough, but typhoid fever had been added.

In the 1922/23 annual report, the Medical Superintendent noted that although admissions had been very light in the early part of that year, a measles epidemic had raged between March and June 1923. The new measles ward pavilions had opened just in time: Scholes noting that if their erection had been delayed another twelve months, a vast amount of suffering and considerable loss of life would have occurred. There was also an outbreak of influenza in June 1923 (90 patients admitted). In regards to these two illnesses the only patients admitted were those suffering from 'complications'—broncho-pneumonia or gastroenteritis, for example. Scholes drew attention to the fact that staffing levels were well up to strength throughout the year but noted that influenza and rubella (which had not occurred in Melbourne for some years) had taken a heavy toll on nursing staff, with 29 nurses being off-duty due to illness at one time. On a brighter note he was pleased to record that the hospital's overall mortality rate of 1.93 per cent was the lowest in the history of the hospital and that, if deaths which occurred within

Whooping cough (pertussis) is a severe, sometimes fatal, infectious disease caused by the colonisation of the air passages by the bacterium *Bordetella pertussis*. The primary symptom is, as the name suggests, violent coughing associated with a sharp intake of breath that causes the characteristic 'whoop'. People become infected by inhaling contaminated droplets from coughs and sneezes. Cerebral hypoxia, bronchopneumonia and secondary pneumonia are possible complications. A small proportion of babies die due to hypoxia, but infection in adults may be mild or even asymptomatic. Whooping cough was first clearly described by de Baillou in Paris in 1578. The name 'pertussis' was given about a hundred years later, by Sydenham in England, but the disease was also called 'chincough', and 'slime cough' (due to the clear sticky mucus produced). The causative organism was isolated at the Pasteur Institute in 1906, by Bordet and Gengou, and named Bordet-Gengou bacteria. Eventually, the name was changed to *Bordetella pertussis*.

The disease was first reported in New South Wales in 1828, brought by passengers on the convict ship *Morley*. Unfortunately the ship was quarantined too late—many people in the colony were infected and several children died. The disease was apparently introduced to Western Australia in the 1940s by the 21st Regiment, with tragic consequences for local Aborigines. By 1848 whooping cough was endemic in Western Australia and probably was well established in Victoria by 1849. A series of epidemics followed its introduction, at intervals of three to four years, with fatalities occurring mainly in children under five. The National Health and Medical Research Council of Australia recommends that babies be immunised against whooping cough from two months of age.

24 hours of admission (15) were deducted, the mortality rate was reduced to 1.57 per cent.

As well as being timely in regards coping with the measles epidemic, the new pavilions were considered a significant improvement in ward design:

> The arrangements of wards in these pavilions has proved a great success. The double H block as suggested is undoubtedly more efficient and much easier to work than the single H block erected in 1915. There is now isolation

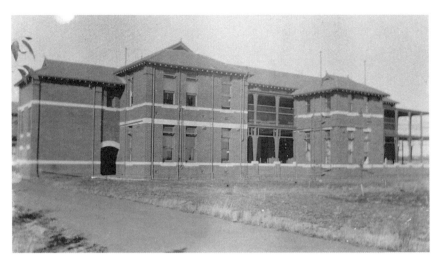

Wards 15 and 16 in the 1920s.

accommodation for about 150 patients, or about a quarter of the total hospital accommodation. In the absence of measles and whooping cough this is ample, but I am of the opinion that in the event of any further extension or replacement of ward accommodation, forty per cent should be set aside for isolation purposes.

The *Nurses' Act* passed in 1923 had a considerable impact on the hospital. The Act established the Nurses' Board and invested it with authority over all matters pertaining to training standards and registration of nurses. Previously these matters had been controlled by the Royal Victorian Trained Nurses' Association, which had been established in 1901. This association later became the Royal Victorian College of Nursing. While still on a nursing theme we might mention that 1923 also saw a croquet green constructed in the hospital grounds for use of the nursing staff. A sign of continuity in the hospital was seen when in 1924 Sir George Cuscaden MD was elected as chair of the Board. Cuscaden had been a member of the original committee formed in 1897 for the Queen's Memorial Fund.

The original motor ambulance cars of the hospital were replaced during the year with Dodge chassis, the bodies being transferred to the new chassis. Three of the old chassis were sold but one was retained for conversion into a motor wagon for market expeditions and for transporting female staff to Clifton Hill—this previously being done by horse wagon.

Scholes summarises the disease patterns for 1923/24:

A quiet Spring and Summer were once again followed by a very busy Autumn, the number of occupied beds rising from 160 in January to 600 in May.

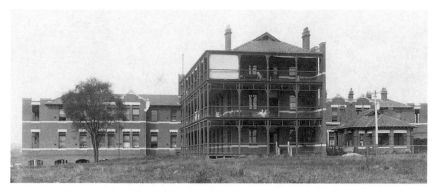

The nurses home in the early 1920s.

Scarlet fever was more active than usual during the autumn, and as it subsided, there began the most severe and extensive epidemic of whooping cough that Melbourne has experienced for many years. Its prevalence was first noted in May.

The epidemics of measles and rubella died out in the Spring of 1923. During their course of a few months 417 patients with measles and 357 with rubella, were admitted to hospital. Diphtheria was not so prevalent as in recent years. The peak appears to have been reached in 1918.

What a world of tragedy and drama Scholes describes. It had, in fact, been a particularly difficult year for the hospital, with 119 patients dying from a total admission of 3929, a mortality rate of 3.07 per cent—well above the previous year's 1.93 per cent. This increase was largely due to a whooping cough epidemic. Whooping cough remained an intransigent killer with a mortality rate of over 25 per cent. An outbreak in Melbourne in May–June 1924 led to 102 whooping cough victims being admitted to Queen's Memorial Hospital. Of these, 25 died, a tragically high number, but this mortality rate of 28.09 per cent was within the normal range for this disease. Scholes noted, somewhat ruefully, that 'Since whooping cough patients were first admitted to the hospital, in no year has the mortality been much lower. Nearly all cases are of very young children with complications.'

The nurses' home (Yarra House) was expanded to the south in 1924/ 25—as recommended by Scholes in the 1923 annual report. Plans for the extension were prepared by the architects Anketell and Henderson, approved by the Board in September 1924, and submitted to the Public Health Department, who accepted the plans with the proviso that two extra bathrooms be incorporated. The amended plans were put out to tender, the winning tender being submitted by W. Hayes. The extension was completed at the end of June 1925.

The usual pattern of admissions occurred in 1924/25, with whooping cough continuing to exact an appalling toll (172 admissions, 45 deaths, mortality rate 24.33 per cent). Diphtheria admissions, however (1605, admissions, 42 deaths, mortality rate 2.56), were the lowest since 1910. In the annual report, Scholes commented on an outbreak of poliomyelitis in the autumn and early winter of 1925:

> Sixteen patients were admitted, of whom three died, and the remaining thirteen were still in hospital on 30th June. These patients needed prolonged and expensive treatment; in addition to the considerable mortality, there is a high percentage of resultant crippling and deformity, and it is hoped that the threatened epidemic next winter will not eventuate.

Scholes' fears of a polio epidemic were to prove all too well founded over the next few years.

It was noted in the 1924/25 annual report in 1925 that the hospital's four ambulance cars had travelled a grand total of 40 509 miles, there being 2900 separate trips to bring 3807 patients to the hospital. The hospital had come a long way from 1903 when it had been forced to borrow a horse because it had no form of transport of its own.

Dr M. T. MacEachern (Associate Director of the American College of Surgeons), an expert on hospitals and hospital design, visited the hospital in January 1926. In his report to the state government he wrote that 'In Melbourne the size of the City warrants a large separate institution of high grade for infectious cases. The Queen's Memorial Infectious Diseases hospital, Melbourne, is one of the best, if not the best, from the standpoints of physical plant and management, which I have ever seen.' To receive such a glowing report from a noted authority on hospitals was a most welcome and fitting tribute to the high standards of medical and nursing care, management and physical facilities that the hospital provided.

During the summer of 1926 the Children's Hospital in Melbourne, overtaxed due to the prevalence of infantile diarrhoea, asked Queen's Memorial Hospital to admit a number of patients. In providing this assistance, Queen's Memorial added bacillary and amoebic dysentery to the list of diseases which it could treat. During the year the Royal Australian Air Force took an aerial photograph of the hospital and presented it with copies. The Board noted in its report how appreciative the hospital was of this courtesy. The 1926/27 annual report once again focused attention on the problem of attracting nursing staff:

> Owing to the difficulty experienced in obtaining sufficient Nurses to properly staff the wards, consideration was given to pay and working conditions. A new schedule of rates of pay was adopted, which provided for increases by annual

Poliomyelitis (polio, infantile paralysis) is a viral infection of the central nervous system. The virus is common and usually its effects are confined to the throat and intestine—with symptoms somewhat similar to a mild digestive upset or flu. In about 1 per cent of cases, however, the infection has a catastrophic impact and results in paralysis. The disease is life-threatening if the muscles of the chest and throat are affected. Polio has probably affected people for thousands of years. An Egyptian stone engraving over three thousand years old, shows what appears to be a polio victim. A doctor in London in 1784 described a disease which was probably polio, however the first definite clinical description was that of Moneggia in 1813. Landsteiner identified the polio virus in 1908.

The first recorded polio epidemic in Australia occurred in South Australia in 1895. In 1903 and 1904 an extensive outbreak occurred in New South Wales, Victoria, Queensland and South Australia, with a further outbreak in Victoria in 1908. The Salk vaccine was introduced in the 1950s. This contains formalin-inactivated viruses and is given by intramuscular injection. In the early 1960s the Sabin vaccine (OPV: oral poliomyelitis vaccine) was introduced. This contains live attenuated viruses and is more effective, easier to administer and gives longer protection than the Salk vaccine (the disadvantage, however, is that a very small proportion of people develop paralytic poliomyelitis). Vaccination programs have almost eliminated the threat of polio in Australia.

increments, as an inducement to Nurses to remain at the hospital. A maximum of £170 per annum for the highest grade is now attainable after eight years' service. The increased rates were advertised, and brought about a slight improvement, but as the Staff was still short of requirements, it was found necessary to engage a number of trained Nurses, at the ruling rate, during the winter.

The annual report for 1927/1928 recorded a successful campaign for resolving the staffing problem:

The shortage of Nursing Staff, referred to in the last Report, which had compelled the Board to the engagement of a number of Trained Nurses, was still causing concern. A special Committee, appointed to consider the position, recommended that publicity be given to the serious position of the Institution. As a result of this, the Staff was brought up to the required strength. The Board is indebted to the Press and to the management of [radio station] 3LO for their assistance in this direction.

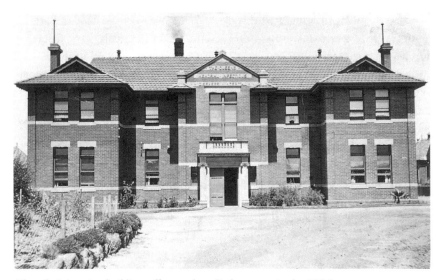

The administration building, offices and medical quarters in the 1920s.

Fifteen cases of poliomyelitis (eight deaths) were recorded in Victoria during 1927, and diphtheria cases rose to 3254 with 93 fatalities. It was particularly unfortunate at this time that a bottle of diphtheria immunising material became contaminated at Bundaberg, Queensland, and caused several deaths. This contamination led to a good deal of fear and renewed distrust of immunisation in the general community. Scarlet fever antitoxin serum was introduced at this time and for two-and-a-half years was given to all cases, but thereafter was only given to the most serious cases. This antitoxin reduced the mortality rate from scarlet fever (sulphonamides, discovered by Gerhard Domagk in 1932, were not introduced until the 1940s by which time the death rate from scarlet fever had already fallen. The 1927/28 annual report noted that the year had brought a 'more severe than usual' type of scarlet fever: without the antitoxic serum, 'The mortality would probably have been doubled or trebled at least, and it is likely also that the incidence of complications would have been higher'. Although pleased to record the very positive impact of the new serum, Scholes presented a rather depressing analysis of infection patterns:

> The incidence of coccal complications has been very high throughout the year. This otitis media [middle ear infection] occurred in 10 per cent of cases, and the abnormal frequency of the less common complications is present throughout the list. This has been noted during the year, not only in scarlatina, but in the other infections also, and the explanation apparently, is that at present we are passing through a period of high streptococcal virulence . . .

It is a sad truth lying at the very heart of our struggle to combat and eradicate disease that for every step forward we take usually have to take a step back, as the infection-causing microbes appear to draw upon their evolutionary cunning and virulent energy to respond to the threat directed towards them. In his 1928/29 report, Scholes reflected on the changing pattern of the hospital's work: 'For many years two seasons or periods could be expected, a busy period (autumn and winter), and a quiet period (spring and summer). This feature is becoming less evident each year, due in part to the increasing variety of diseases admitted.' An outbreak of poliomyelitis occurred between January and June, with 156 cases in Victoria (25 deaths).

The hospital and its patients had reason to be grateful to the media when, as a result of the *Herald* 'Wireless Appeal', a 'large body of men from the Telephone and Railways Telegraph Departments attended and completed in one afternoon an installation extending over the whole of the wards. This has proved a great boon to the patients, who have repeatedly expressed their gratitude for the pleasure afforded.'

Reflecting on the 1920s when he was Deputy Medical Superintendent of the hospital, Dr H. McLorinan recalled many years later that:

> Fairfield, with its able superintendent, Dr Scholes, achieved a considerable international reputation. We may in retrospect be somewhat critical now of some of the methods used; but the fact remains that an amazing amount of work was carried out with, on the whole, excellent results. It was in fever hospitals that most of the work of isolation and barrier nursing techniques were first propounded, and medical asepsis, as we know it, had its origin in fever hospitals.

For the first time in its history the 1928/29 annual report included a section entitled 'Staff Illness'. The statistics presented make startling reading and perhaps to a large extent explain the staffing problems which had plagued the hospital since its earliest days:

> There were 178 instances of sickness among the nursing staff. The large number is partly accounted for by the fact that nurses are required strictly to report any ailment or symptoms, however mild. The majority of illnesses were very mild, and of the 19 cases of diphtheria a large proportion were only technically diphtheria. There were 17 cases of scarlet fever, two of measles, two of rubella, one of whooping cough, one of varicella, and two of mumps.

On a more positive note the report also recorded that Dr Wynne had been employed as a consultant in diseases of the ear, nose and throat in November 1928 and that his work—particularly the many operations he had performed —had been 'very satisfactory indeed'.

The economic depression during the early 1930s led many cost-saving municipal councils to discharge their health inspectors or place them on part-time employment. This was particularly unfortunate and indeed dangerous. The same economic conditions which had tempted local authorities to reduce health care provisions had placed many Victorians in poverty, unable to maintain reasonable standards of diet, clothing or housing—all factors which made them increasingly susceptible to illness and infectious disease.

Scholes choose the beginning of the new decade to reflect in 1930 upon the development of the hospital and his analysis of changing patterns in infectious disease is worth quoting at some length:

> During the past 20 years a gradual change has taken place in the function of this hospital. Originally, the main purpose and idea of isolation hospitals was isolation. It was imagined that if all cases of legally notifiable diseases were isolated (in the case of scarlatina for an arbitrary time), the incidence would be very greatly diminished, if not abolished. Those of us who have been actively engaged in the work have never laboured under any such delusion. The number of reported cases, in this as in other countries, has shown no fall, and in view of the fact that only a certain number of infected persons show symptoms justifying notification and isolation. At the same time, it is believed the isolation hospital has played a great part in the reduction of mortality, and of the serious types of these diseases, by reason of the fact that practically all severe cases of infection presumably by malign strains of bacteria, are isolated and treated in hospital.
>
> The change is that the hospital is to be regarded as a hospital for the treatment of patients who, for one reason or another, cannot be treated in their own homes or in other hospitals rather than for isolation only.
>
> The question then arises as to which classes of patients come under this category. The diseases gazetted as admissible to this hospital are diphtheria, scarlet fever, measles, whooping cough, cerebrospinal meningitis, infantile paralysis, influenza, and dysentery. In addition, a number are actually received of cases of mumps, chickenpox, erysipelas, typhoid fever, and many laryngitis, tonsillitis, and various skin eruptions, sent in with provisional diagnosis of diphtheria or scarlet fever.
>
> It will be conceded generally, that nearly all cases of mumps, chickenpox, measles influenza, and whooping cough can receive adequate treatment in their homes, and that admissions to hospital should be reserved for special cases, where complications are present or threatened, or where home conditions do not permit of proper care.
>
> This is very true, but I would be inclined to make an exception in the case of measles in poorer homes. The results of treatment of early measles is so very good, and the development of bronchopneumonia and other complications so rare, that it would pay the community handsomely to treat all cases of early measles from poor homes, in hospital. The results in whooping cough are not nearly so good, and admission should be strictly reserved.
>
> I have found that few medical men will take responsibility of treating diphtheria patients at home, save in special circumstances. We may assume that admission will generally be sought for cases of this disease.

Scholes was particularly concerned about scarlet fever and its complications:

> Scarlet fever presents by far the most difficult problem. This disease has changed in character of late years. In this country there has been no epidemic of a really severe form for a generation or more; nevertheless each year there have been a few toxic cases, the vast majority of the remainder being mild. In 1927 I noted the beginnings of another change, and have commented on it in Annual Reports since. Complications, reinfections, and relapses have become so common in originally mild infections, that nowadays no case can safely be labelled as mild till convalescence is quite complete and infection disappeared. Various causes can be suggested—the coming into contact with secondary strains of germs from other patients in convalescence, the administration of serum producing an artificial immunity instead of allowing the patient to develop it for himself, a mutual tolerance between bacterium and patient, allowing the free development of the septic processes, and so on. The fact remains, that mild scarlet fever is a much more dangerous disease than moderately severe diphtheria in hospital. I have taken pains during the last few years to find out all I can about the results in scarlet fever treated at home, and I conclude that the same condition of affairs exists. While profoundly dissatisfied with the results of treatment of mild scarlet fever in hospital, I confess I am not sure of what consequences would arise should a very large proportion of patients be treated at home.

This was not, of course, merely academic speculation, as it had considerable relevance to hospital policy in selecting and restricting admissions. Scholes' underlying concern was the bed occupancy rates: 'For the greater part of the year under review, every ward was occupied, and it is obvious that Fairfield cannot cope with an epidemic, either of diphtheria or scarlatina. Should one occur, restriction or selection of patients for admission will be necessary.' In a general hospital and most specialist hospitals it is generally held that the higher the bed occupancy rate the more effective the hospital. In an

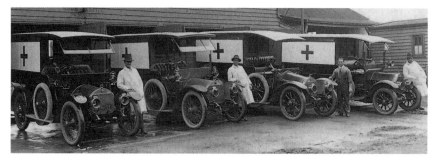

A fleet of ambulances with attendants in the 1930s; note that they do not carry the hospital's name, because of the stigma attached to infectious disease.

infectious diseases hospital, on the other hand, a consistently high occupancy rate means that the hospital is not in a position to provide an immediate response to any sudden epidemics which might arise and thus in effect is not able to use its expert staff and specialised facilities when the community most needs them.

It is clear that a good deal of thought was being given to the role and structure of the hospital at this time. Thus Scholes at the request of the Board prepared a report on the 'reorganisation of medical staff'. As a result of this report the Board decided to establish a small permanent staff which could be supplemented when required. A number of temporary junior medical officers were appointed on 1 July 1930, including a Deputy Medical Superintendent, Pathologist, Bacteriologist, Second Resident Medical Officer and Third Resident Medical Officer. It was considered that

> during quiet periods, and for a limited time, during which it may be impossible to obtain a full staff, the work of the hospital can be carried out efficiently by the above resident officers. A complete reorganisation of duties is being made, which should make for efficiency and economy, and it is hoped that by the establishment of an experienced Staff, many minor reforms and improvements can be brought about.

Illnesses amongst the nursing staff again loomed large in the 1929/30 annual report. Of the more serious cases among the 193 recorded instances of nursing staff illness there were 27 cases of diphtheria, 24 of scarlet fever, 4 of measles, 1 of rubella, 2 of varicella, 1 of pleurisy and 1 of tuberculosis. Tragically, one of the nurses who caught diphtheria died from the illness. She had paid the highest possible price for her commitment to a caring profession and her death reminds us of the dangers that hospital staff faced on a daily basis.

The then highest number of admissions in its history occurred in 1930/ 31, when the hospital admitted 4954 patients. As a result, however, on 2 April 1931 the hospital was forced to restrict admissions. All medical practitioners were asked to stop sending mild cases of infectious disease to the hospital and to treat patients who could be isolated at home themselves. Despite this measure the hospital became 'dangerously overcrowded', with over 2000 patients being admitted during March–June. The great danger of overcrowding and overworked staff was, of course, cross-infection, and medical staff were acutely conscious that conditions within the hospital were creating an environment where cross-infection was becoming increasingly likely. On 22 June the hospital could no longer cope with the number of patients under care and was forced to reduce the number of occupied beds by about 100. In part the problems had related to sudden increases in diphtheria and scarlet fever in March 1931. Scholes had foreseen that an epidemic of either of these

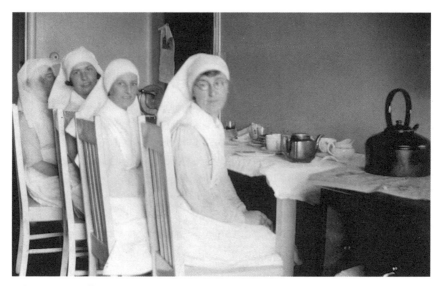

The nursing staff always took morning tea, usually prepared by the junior nurses on duty, in the ward pantry. Here, in the 1930s, they face the wall.

diseases would force the hospital to adopt a policy of restriction or selection of patients, and his fears were now realised. As well as restricting admissions, the hospital was forced into the 'discharge of many patients as soon as they were physically well, without bacteriological examination'—clearly an unhealthy state of affairs. Scholes was pessimistic about the hospital's ability to cope with the demands made upon it .'It may be taken for granted that a certain amount of restriction of admissions must continue during the summer, and unless or until further accommodation is provided, a large proportion of patients will not be able to be received for treatment after March next.'

In light of the difficulty in admitting those who needed hospitalisation, the Board acted quickly on Scholes' urgings. Early in 1932 a deputation from the Board waited upon the Minister, and requested the extension of the hospital, which was then dangerously overcrowded and inadequate to meet the demand for admission, many patients being turned away daily. The Minister suggested using the buildings in different districts, but these, after inspection, were found unsuitable for the work, and would have required a separate overhead, involving great expense. The government then authorised the erection of one '"H" type Wards Block of 50 beds, to be proceeded with immediately, at an estimated cost of £10,000, including the furniture and equipment'. The foundation stone for the new ward block was laid on 30 November 1932. An increase of fifty beds could not, of course, resolve the accommodation problem, but it gave the hospital greater flexibility and allowed better grouping and isolation of patients. The building was opened in August 1933 by Sir Stanley Argyle, Premier of Victoria and Minister for Health. This addition brought the number of beds in the hospital to 720. Plans were also put in place for another expansion to the nurses home, which had been extended only eight years earlier. The new extension, at a cost of £25 000, was designed by A. and K. Henderson in a style which matched the earlier buildings.

Scholes described 1931/32 as 'a very trying year.' Total admissions for the year (5947) exceeded the previous year's record admissions by 993, about 20 per cent. Impressive as this increase is, it would have been much higher if the hospital had been in a position to admit all patients referred to it for treatment. In his summary of the year, Scholes—who was himself in poor health —presented a blunt and uncompromising account of the problems which had beset the hospital:

> For the greater part of the year admissions were restricted to those actually ill and in need of nursing and medical care, and for short periods to those certified as dangerously or seriously ill. In view of the repeated warnings given over a period of years, and the efforts made by the Board to secure increased accommodation, the blame for the deplorable state of affairs which existed for the whole year cannot be laid at the door of the Board. Under the circumstances the results obtained, so far as saving life was concerned, were wonderfully good, and considering the class of case admitted, the mortality percentages of diphtheria and scarlet fever can only be described as amazing. The incidence of complications and toxic effects, however was very high … One bad feature of the overcrowding was the frequency of cross-infections, particularly in the spring months. The principal manifestation was the infection of patients by haemolytic streptococci. For several years past, beginning with 1928, I had drawn attention in annual reports to the increasing number of carriers of streptococci in the Community. During certain periods of the year under review a large percentage of all children admitted were found to be carrying or to be infected with haemolytic streptococci. They were responsible for a fair amount of disease outside, but in attacking susceptible diphtheria and scarlet fever convalescents they did far more damage. Fortunately we had been expecting the invasion for some years, and early and energetic serum treatment undoubtedly saved many lives. There was rather more cross-infection by diphtheria than usual, but without any bad effects, and no deaths. Measles, mumps, whooping cough, and chickenpox were moderately prevalent at various times, and gave rise to a certain amount of cross-infection. Had proper accommodation been available, most of this could have been avoided … The daily average number of occupied beds was 508, the highest on record. Of course it was kept at a more or less artificial level, and had accommodation been available would probably have been very much higher … Staff illness again showed a gratifying decrease, but I regret to report the death of a nurse from septicaemia …

Despite the huge pressure upon him as Medical Superintendent of a grossly overstrained and under-resourced hospital and his own poor health. Scholes still managed to turn his inquiring and incisive mind to changes and reforms in infectious disease medicine which were indicated by the emergency measures he had been forced to implement:

> In order to make room for sick persons requiring treatment, it became necessary at times to discharge a number of persons who had recovered very well, but without the routine procedure of obtaining negative swabs previously. The relative number of return cases was not very appreciably increased, and in an ordinary year might not have been increased at all. I am of the opinion, as previously expressed, that the prescribed practice of requiring two negative swabs before discharge of diphtheria patients could be modified to advantage.
>
> The time is now ripe also to suggest the abandonment of the routine disinfectant bath immediately before discharge of patients and the discouragement of the admission to hospital of healthy diphtheria carriers, excepting in special cases and in inter-epidemic periods. I am quite aware that popular opinion, and also what might be called popular medical opinion, supports the continuance of these practices, but expert opinion throughout the world is inclining to the view that they are unnecessary and often unwise, and I cordially agree with this.

Scholes, who had been overworked for many years and had been suffering from ill health for some time, was granted nine months leave of absence in March 1933, to undertake extensive investigations on the operations of fever hospitals overseas and in particular to study the latest methods of hospital administration in other countries. Dr Henry McLorinan, Deputy Medical Superintendent, who had worked at the hospital since 1920, was appointed acting Medical Superintendent in Scholes' absence.

The 1932/33 annual report, as part of a discussion on cross-infection and infections, reproduces a letter of instructions given to patients' relatives on a patient's discharge from the hospital. This letter, which tends to assume a middle-class level of income and housing, placed a good deal of responsibility on the people caring for the discharged patient:

> 1. In scarlet fever, and to a lesser extent in diphtheria, no means exist of enabling us to state with positive certainty that any individual child is no longer infectious, liable to recurrence, or free from the risk of late affects. Tests and swabs are not absolutely reliable, and also many children though not infectious on discharge, become infected again almost at once on mixing with other persons. You are therefore advised to keep the patient away from other children as much as possible during the next fortnight or so, and all direct contact such as kissing, sleeping in the same bed, and overcrowding should be avoided. In the event of sore throat, discharge from the nose or ear, swollen glands in the neck, or other untoward signs, you should consult your doctor at once.

2. During convalescence from diphtheria, fatigue or over exertion should be avoided, and any of the following symptoms should be carefully noted, viz., dragging of the feet, a nasal tone of the voice, or food returning through the nostrils. If any of these conditions occur, medical attention should be immediately obtained.
3. A short holiday in the country, if the weather be suitable, is always desirable during convalescence.
4. Discharged patients should be warmly clothed and otherwise protected from cold.

As a response to high cross-infection rates, McLorinan produced a report on the subject and the report was considered important enough to include in the annual report. It presents a clear and immediate picture of the hospital's daily operations and continuing battle against infectious disease:

> Last year's figures show that during the year a little over 4 per cent. of cases, while in hospital, developed some other infectious complaint. Last year, owing to the persistent overcrowding and inability to close or quarantine any of the wards, was the worst in the history, as records cross-infection.
>
> This figure, at first glance, may seem high. Let us look at the question from my point of view. The average duration of a child's stay in this hospital is about one month. Now, if these children were running about the suburbs instead of in hospital for that time, I would venture to state that considerably more than 4 per cent would contract some infectious disease. From this point of view, the percentage would be somewhat re-assuring. It is a common idea among the public generally, that any disease contracted by a patient in a fever hospital must be caused by carelessness, and that it has been carried by an attendant from another ward. Actually this rarely happens, and I might almost say, *never* happens. Practically all the trouble is caused by patients being admitted into a ward while they are in the incubation stage of the disease.
>
> All the common infectious diseases have an incubation period. This is the quiescent period of the disease between the time of actual contact with the disease and the time when the first symptoms develop. During this quiet period there are no symptoms, and no authority on earth can say that this child is going to develop the disease.
>
> Now, children are admitted to hospital in the quiet period of the disease, and in due course, infect a number of children in the ward. This ward has now to be closed to admissions and in spite of all precautions, it is considered fortunate, if less than a dozen children become infected from this case.
>
> The commonest of the cross-infections in this hospital is chicken-pox. This is highly infectious and is difficult to eradicate from a ward. Fortunately, the results are never serious. Diphtheria is fairly common in scarlet fever wards. It is so well known that convalescent scarlet fever patients are liable to develop diphtheria, not only in hospital, but also in cases nursed at home, that Medical Text Books frequently refer to Post Scarlatinal Diphtheria. The cases, however, are almost

always mild . . . These patients do, however, have a longer stay in hospital. I have never seen a fatal case of diphtheria occur in a scarlet fever ward during the last ten years at Fairfield.

Scarlet fever occurring in diphtheria wards is one of the most dreaded by fever hospitals. Scarlet fever is caused by a germ known as the Haemolytic Streptococcus. This germ may be cause in some people true scarlet fever, and in others septic throats. During the last two years in Melbourne, septic throats were very prevalent and a large proportion of them were caused by this germ. Consequently scarlet fever carriers became very numerous in Melbourne, and it is very difficult to detect these carriers until after they have caused an outbreak in a ward.

Measles, whooping cough, and mumps, do not as a rule cause much trouble. In all cases, the parents are told that such things are not the fault of the hospital. Also a circular letter was sent to all contributory councils on the question of return cases. This briefly explained that a small percentage of cases discharged from the hospital will always be likely to infect others, in spite of the fact that a personal examination was made, in that swab tests were all negative before discharge . . .

Matron E. M. Walker celebrated twenty-five years continuous service at the hospital in 1934—an achievement which was marked by celebrations.

Given the long history of overcrowding and intense pressure, it was no doubt with a sigh of relief that Scholes—returned from his sabbatical—was able to record in the 1933/34 annual report that for the first time since 1929, a whole year went by with no overcrowding—due to increased flexibility given by the six new wards. The greater number of self-contained units reduced cross-infection and, for the first time since 1929/30, it had not been necessary to restrict patient admission. The daily average number of occupied beds was 468, compared with 534 for the previous year. The decrease was partly due to the lower number of admissions, and partly to a reduction in the average stay of patients.

One commentator has suggested that these lower admission rates marked the beginning of 'the sharp decline in the incidence of infectious disease admissions'.[5] Whether this was indeed a turning point in the incidence of infectious disease or not, it certainly marked a welcome relief for the hospital. The depression years had brought great difficulty and hardship for the hospital, as for the community as a whole. Given the financial restrictions then in place, the hospital did remarkably well to obtain funding for significant additions and to emerge from the depression years stronger than ever. In keeping with the sense of optimism and confidence about the future that was felt around the hospital at this time, the Board decided to erect and equip a new laboratory in the next financial year.

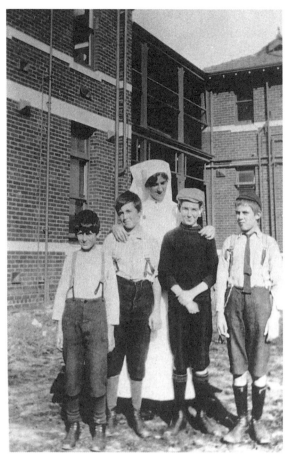

Young patients 'well on the way to recovery' in the 1930s.

The pattern of lower admissions continued into the following year, which Scholes described as 'a quiet one'. Admission numbers (4552) were the lowest since 1929/30 and a massive 1495 below the 1931/32 record. Cross-infection of specific infectious diseases in the wards was infrequent, but there were other problems:

> an unusually large number of patients were admitted while incubating a second and in some cases a third disease, and the number of patients found on admission to be carrying haemolytic streptococci or diphtheria bacilli, while suffering from other diseases, was high. These factors necessitated the adjustment or closing of ward after ward, almost incessantly throughout the year. In this connection the subdivisible wards have been of great value.

While scarlet fever and diphtheria numbers were well down, measles, influenza and whooping cough rates remained high. The reduction of scarlet fever admissions took a lot of pressure off hospital beds as this illness required much longer hospitalisation than the other common infectious diseases. As was his custom, Scholes not only recorded a factual description of the hospital's activities in his yearly report but also presented his thoughts regarding specific treatment patterns. In this instance his focus was on scarlet fever and measles:

> The convalescent period of scarlatina presents the greatest problem in the internal work of a fever hospital, and, in my opinion, is still its most unsatisfactory feature. While the public still believe, and in some cases are even told by their medical advisers that scarlatinal patients are infectious for a fixed period of six weeks, it is difficult for the hospital to take the initiative and run the risk of incurring blame for return cases and the late complications which occur in any event. The fact is that for very many patients the optimum time for discharge from hospital is about the end of the third week. A reasonable period of semi-isolation and occasional medical supervision at home would be necessary, or at least advisable, but I am strongly of opinion that the mass results would be better. It is hoped that general medical and public opinion will some day become educated to the definitely proved facts that there is no fixed period of infectivity of scarlatina, that the period varies both in time and degree, within very wide limits, that a child is quite as likely to be an 'infecting case' if discharged from hospital after three months as after three weeks, and while the human body and haemolytic streptococci remain as they are, 'return' and 'infecting' cases will continue to occur. A more rational attitude, and a more rational procedure carried into effect, would save both money and health.

Scholes was positive about the advantages of treating selected cases of measles in hospital:

> This is a lifesaving measure, and should be extended so that no young child in a poor home, or in need of hospital treatment, should be denied it. The worst complications of measles are preventable, and have been efficiently prevented in this hospital for the past twenty years. The recovery rate of those admitted to hospital with dangerous complications has been very good also.

He was clearly optimistic about scarlet fever and measles, but his tone changed when he turned to that great scourge, whooping cough: 'The treatment of selected and complicated cases of whooping cough in hospital is a matter of necessity, not of choice. The results are to be regarded as satisfactory, and no more. The case fatality in this hospital has varied from 15 to 32 per cent., and this year is 21.4.' Clearly the desperately high fatality rate for whooping cough victims and the inability of medical science to intervene

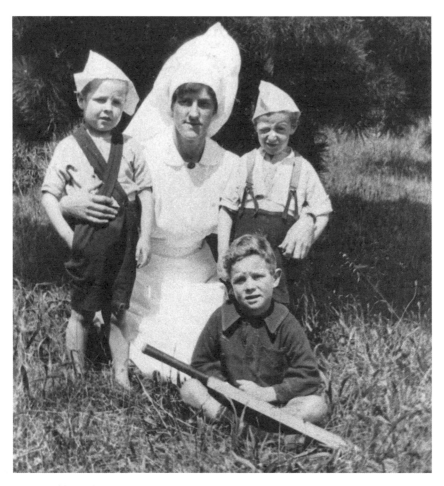

*These children, playing with a nurse in the hospital gardens in the 1930s, are recovering
from diphtheria and scarlet fever. They are allowed to wear their own clothes while
awaiting three negative ear, nose and throat swabs.*

effectively had dispirited even such an experienced infectious disease specialist as Scholes.

On a brighter note Scholes' report was able to boast the opening of the
new, fully equipped laboratory at the hospital during the autumn and to note
that it was already doing excellent work. As well as performing routine examinations the laboratory was also able to undertake, albeit in a small way, some
research work. This critical aspect of the hospital's work was, as we shall see,
an area that would expand dramatically in the following years.

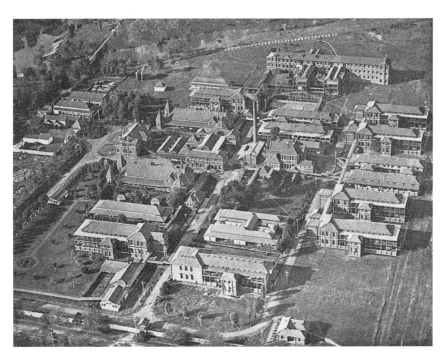

An aerial photograph of the hospital, 1934.

In a display of foresight, the hospital purchased a Drinker Respirator, or 'iron lung', in 1936. The respirator, imported from London, was installed in one of the four receiving houses, which was especially converted for this purpose. The hospital had recognised the need for such a machine for some time: indeed, in the three month prior to its installation four children suffering from respiratory paralysis had been transferred to the Children's Hospital for treatment. The respirator was a great success: 'In the three months following the installation of our machine three children were treated in it, recovery following in two of them. Of all the seven children, four recovered and the average duration of stay in the machine for these four was about twelve days. It has paid for itself.' As we shall shortly see, the purchase of this respirator was to prove most timely.

During the first seven months of the 1935/36 financial year, the hospital was quiet, with no serious disease outbreaks and no particular illness being prevalent. This was a lull before the storm, for between February and May the hospital was inundated with diphtheria patients. For a variety of reasons this outbreak, which saw an astonishing 3555 diphtheria admissions, was a particularly unusual and interesting one. Scholes was clearly fascinated by the epidemic:

> The most remarkable feature of the year was the great autumnal wave of diph-
> theria. The second was its very low fatality, the lowest on record [55 deaths,
> mortality rate 1.57 per cent]. It is possible almost to indicate the actual dates of
> its beginning and end, and to say that it began on 12th February and ended on
> 30th May. The autumnal wave is a well marked character of diphtheria in
> Melbourne, but, in 27 years, I have never seen such a curious explosion. The low
> fatality was due, in my opinion, to two causes:–
> (1) The publicity given to the prevalence of the disease. This resulted in patients
> being sent in at an earlier stage of the disease than usual. During the epidemic
> period, the average duration of illness before admission was a fraction under two
> days, instead of nearly three days. The 'scare' did not result in a larger proportion
> than usual of patients being admitted not suffering from diphtheria. On the
> contrary, the proportion ultimately recorded as 'tonsillitis', 'laryngitis', etc., was
> lower than usual. The publicity given was justified by results, and was the cause,
> in my opinion, of a large saving of life.
> (2) The fact before mentioned that during the outbreak, or, at any rate, till late
> in May, there was a singular absence of streptococcal element in the diphtheria
> cases. Not only were ordinary coccal complications such as otitis [ear infection],
> rare, but also gross sepsis; and fulminating strepto-diphtheria was hardly
> seen. There was plenty of pure diphtheria of a malignant and toxic nature
> though the majority of cases were moderate or mild. From the incomplete data
> available, it is not possible to find any unusual prevalence of a particular type of
> diphtheria bacillus. A large number of cases, taken at random by Dr Kelsey,
> showed all forms to be present in the epidemic, gravis, mitis, and intermedius.

As epidemics go this one was—from the hospital's point of view—relatively benign and unproblematic. The coming year was to present an epidemic of a different order. The year 1936/37 was a most unusual one in the history of the hospital. The diphtheria epidemic which, based on many years' experience, was expected in March 1937 did not arise; and amazingly there were only four admissions for measles—each of these cases was 'exotic' in as much as they had been imported from outside the state. Writing in December 1937, Scholes noted that 'for nearly two years there has been no case of measles arising in Melbourne' and put this statistic in historical context: 'To my knowledge, never during the past thirty years has Melbourne enjoyed a freedom from this disease for more than a few months'. With both diphtheria and measles admissions dramatically lower than expected, the hospital for most of the year was 'rather overstaffed'. In May a recurrence of rubella (34 admissions) which had not been seen in Melbourne for fourteen years, provided further confirmation of the wild and unpredictable nature of infectious diseases.

In his annual report, Scholes argued forcibly that the hospital urgently required a program of works to remodel and extend the administration block; rebuild the hospital's garages, workshops and men's quarters; remodel some of the ward pavilions; and last, but by no means least, demolish Ward 3—the last of the old wooden wards—and construct a new isolation pavilion on its site.

The 'overstaffing' resulting from the unusual disease patterns in 1936/37 was to prove useful when an 'unprecedentedly severe epidemic of polio-myelitis' descended upon Victoria in July 1937. The hospital was, of course, at the centre of the poliomyelitis emergency. From 25 July it admitted all cases from the metropolitan and central country areas of Victoria. Scholes as well as leading the effort to provide treatment and care for poliomyelitis victims, was also a member of the Consultative Council, Aftercare Committee and Research Committee set up in response to the epidemic. The demands on him during the early months of the polio epidemic are well illustrated by the fact that it was 30 December before he found time to write his report for the pre-vious year's annual report. In explaining the delay, Scholes simply stated: 'much of my time was taken up by matters which were regarded as more urgent'.

The epidemic of poliomyelitis began in the southern suburbs of Mel-bourne in June 1937, later spreading to all parts of the state. By the end of the year there were 1367 recorded cases (1275 cases were admitted to Queen's Memorial Hospital in 1937/38, and 77 of these patients died). The govern-ment appointed a Consultative Council for Poliomyelitis on 22 July which circulated special advice on poliomyelitis; this information was widely dis-seminated through the Health Department, the Education Department and the media. Respirator equipment was situated at 'strategic points' and hospi-tal committees throughout Victoria were involved in coping with the epi-demic. The government appointed a Poliomyelitis After-Care Committee to help organise care for the growing number of poliomyelitis victims. Descend-ing on the community at a time when most other infectious diseases were on the decline, poliomyelitis was to become one of Victoria's main public health problems. Poliomyelitis can be likened to the earlier bubonic plague and the contemporary AIDS epidemic in terms of the feelings of terror and helpless-ness that it inspired in the community. The extent of the problem can be seen from the fact that of 2096 cases had occurred in 1937/38, with 108 deaths. These bald figures mask personal and family tragedy and loss on a vast scale.

In his yearly report (the publication of which was again much delayed due to pressure of work) in 1938, Scholes gives a graphic account of how the hospital coped with the poliomyelitis epidemic:

> The hospital year began quietly, with the prevalence of Diphtheria and Scarlet Fever rather lower than is usual during July. Whooping Cough cases were few,

and Measles had been completely absent from Melbourne for more than a year. An epidemic of Rubella, the first in Melbourne in fourteen years, was at its height, but on account of the mildness of this disease there was no great call on hospital beds. Consequently, it was possible at once to set aside ward blocks for Poliomyelitis as fast as the necessary nursing and staff adjustments could be made, and block after block was opened and staffed until nine ward blocks, accommodating 230 patients, were taken over for this disease . . . The incidence of Diphtheria and Scarlet Fever fell rapidly in September, and admissions were abnormally low for the remainder of the period under review. But the work on all wards was heavy. Not only were the majority of the older and more experienced nurses required for the Poliomyelitis wards, in which, particularly in the respirator wards, a large staff had to be maintained, but very careful nursing and isolation measures were necessary in the Diphtheria and Scarlet Fever wards to prevent infection there. Finally, several hundred patients were admitted as suspected cases of Poliomyelitis, found actually to be suffering from a wide variety of diseases, and for many months, all the isolation accommodation in the hospital was taken up.

Before the epidemic, the hospital had just one Drinker respirator, and late in July two wooden respirators were installed. As the epidemic increased, more respirators were acquired, until the hospital had twenty-three in constant use. At one time, these respirators were being used for 47 patients. The later models were lighter and of simpler construction. Professor Burstall of the Public Health Department, and the firms manufacturing and supplying the various units, assisted in supplying these improved respirators. But by 30 June

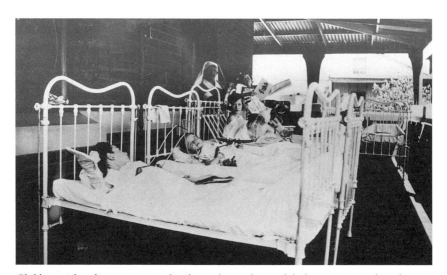

Children with polio are accommodated on a hospital verandah due to overcrowding during the 1937 epidemic.

1938 only 26 patients remained in the poliomyelitis wards—76 had died at the hospital, and the rest had been discharged or transferred to after-care.

If any doubts remained about the necessity for having a specialised infectious diseases hospital to serve the state, the hospital's response to the poliomyelitis emergency must surely have put them to rest. The hospital was able to respond immediately and effectively to the emergency, demonstrating its experience and expertise in treating infectious diseases and its willingness to improvise solutions to the many problems associated with the epidemic. For example, nineteen respirators were produced in the hospital's own workshops,[6] and one of the hospital's ambulances was lined with spongy rubber to assist in the transport of batches of children.

Although Scholes' 1937/38 report focused on poliomyelitis, he did comment on other significant developments during the year and reflected on areas of patient treatment and care that needed improvement:

> Only 17 deaths occurred from Diphtheria, and 3 from Scarlet Fever, during the twelve months. These are by far the lowest figures since the early days of the hospital, a generation back, when it was a very small institution. One factor, of course, was the unusually low number of admissions, but the case fatality figures were also very low. I consider that the hospital treatment of these diseases *during the first fortnight* is now nearly perfect, but that the succeeding weeks, especially in walking convalescents, present many unsatisfactory features. It is to the remedying of these that our future efforts must be directed.

E. M. Walker, who had been Matron since August 1909, died in November 1938. Scholes, who had come to the hospital only the year after her appointment, paid a handsome tribute to her work and character in the 1938/39 annual report:

> It is with great regret that I have to record the death, in November of Miss E. M. Walker, Matron of the hospital. Miss Walker took up duty as Sister-in charge of Diphtheria wards in 1908, and as Matron in August, 1909. From that date until her death, I had the honour of continuous association with her in the hospital, and no tribute that I can pay can do justice to her work and its effects. She was a woman of great courage, personality and ability, and was at her best when the hospital was in difficulty. Particularly I would like to mention the hard and trying years 1911–15, and the period of re-building that followed, and the period of epidemic waves which ended in 1921. The illness which caused her death had been present intermittently for some years and during that time Miss E. V. Watson, the Assistant Matron had many calls made upon her. Miss Watson was Acting Matron until the appointment of Miss Burbidge as Matron in March.

A number of Matron Walker's friends and colleagues erected a sundial in the hospital grounds in her memory in 1941. The same year saw the retirement of A. A. Marsden, who had served the hospital with distinction as secretary since 1915. N. W. Neep was appointed to replace Marsden and served from 1939 to 1940. Another stalwart ended direct involvement with the hospital in July 1941: Evelyn Conyers, the first Matron of the hospital, resigned from the Board after many years of service. Conyers had a record of distinguished service to the nursing profession and during World War I had been appointed Matron-in-Chief of Nursing Services. Her position on the Board was filled by Dr Marion B. Wanliss.

G. N. Burbidge, DipN (Lond), A R San I, took up her duties as Matron on 26 March 1939. At the time of her appointment she was probably the best qualified nurse in Australia, having done post-graduate studies at Great Ormond Street and St Thomas's Hospital, King's College, London University, and been awarded a Diploma in Nursing—at that time unique in Australia. This year also saw Scholes, and by association the hospital, honoured when he was awarded the CMG.

The hitherto poor wages and working conditions of the hospital's nurses were significantly improved on 1 December 1938 when the Nurses' Wages Board conditions came into effect. These new conditions increased wage levels and reduced working hours. The new award of service increased the hospital's total annual payments to nurses by £5400.

The 1938/39 annual report broke with tradition by including illustrations: the aerial photograph of the hospital taken by the Royal Australian Air Force in 1934 and an accompanying plan to explain the functions of the buildings in the photograph. These illustrations remained a regular feature of the hospital's annual reports for many years.

That year was a relatively quiet one for the hospital. Total admissions were fairly low at 3778 and the fatality rate of 1.34 per cent was the lowest in its history. The main features of admission patterns were the steady rise of scarlet fever (1622 admissions), the continued fall in diphtheria (from a decade high level of 3555 in 1936 to 888 in 1939) and the reappearance of measles which had been absent for two and a half years (only 200 admissions but an estimated 40 000–50 000 cases in Melbourne). Although admission levels had been relatively low, the great variety of diseases meant that nearly all of the wards were occupied continuously. The fact that a significant numbers of patients were suffering from three of the 'long incubation period' diseases—measles, rubella and varicella—meant that the possibility of cross-infection was a major concern throughout the year. Fortunately, due to good nursing and patient management, cross-infections were 'few and slight'.

The reputation and status of the hospital and the exceptional qualifications of its new Matron were recognised in 1940 when the Nurses' Board approved the hospital as a training school for nurses and arranged that Queen's Memorial affiliate, for training purposes, with the Alfred, St Vincent's and other hospitals. As part of this new development the hospital appointed a sister tutor, and Ward 8 was equipped as a teaching unit.

World War II had a dramatic impact on the hospital. In 1940 the Deputy Medical Superintendent, Dr H. McLorinan, enlisted for military service, as did other members of staff and Board members. (McLorinan was to serve with distinction in the Middle East and was mentioned in dispatches for distinguished services. He returned from war service as a Lieutenant-Colonel in November 1941 and resumed his position as Deputy Medical Superintendent.) Scholes was a major in the Australian Army Medical Corps Reserve.

The war affected the hospital in areas other than staffing. It had developed a contingency plan for dealing with the outbreak of war, and in September 1939 this plan was put into immediate effect. A number of wards were set aside for military personnel and were soon full to overflowing. Soldiers (1261), airmen (141) and sailors (19) made up a significant proportion of admissions during the year, helping to raise the number of admissions to 6576 (compared with 3778 in the previous year). The type of infections suffered by military personnel tended to be of a minor nature—measles, rubella, respiratory tract infections, influenza, tonsillitis, bronchitis, bronchopneumonia and mumps being the most common. Given that these patients were almost invariably fit, strong young men, it is hardly surprising that only two 'military patients' died in the hospital. Consequently, the fatality rate of 0.84 per cent (for all admissions during the year) was by a long way the lowest in the history of the hos-

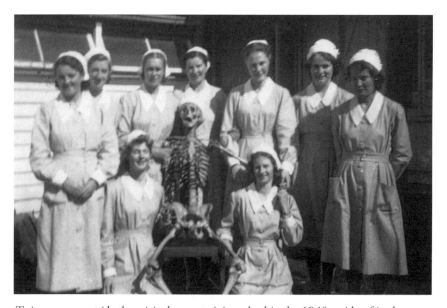

Trainee nurses outside the original nurse training school in the 1940s, with a friend.

pital. Scholes was too honest to make any great claims for this exceptionally low fatality rate, but simply noted that, due to the special circumstances, the figure could not 'be taken seriously for the purposes of comparison'.

A measles epidemic reached its peak in August 1939 and thereafter almost disappeared among the civilian population, but it remained a problem in military camps where it was fed by the constant appearance of new drafts of recruits. Rubella, which reached epidemic proportions in military camps in October, remained a severe problem throughout the year. Commenting on these outbreaks, and in particular on the impact of military service on infectious disease, Scholes drew on his experience as Medical Superintendent of the hospital during World War I:

> Movements and segregation of susceptible young adults from country districts have been responsible not only for the prolongation of prevalence of measles and lighting up of rubella, but also, in my opinion, for the widespread epidemic of upper respiratory tract infection which has affected both civil and military sections of the community. It would appear that the normal virulence of infective agents has been exalted by passage through a large number of susceptible individuals living under new conditions. There has been a reproduction of the picture presented in 1916, of waves of different infectious diseases following one another in quick succession.

Diphtheria, which had been for so many years one of the hospital's greatest problems, had been declining since 1937 and in 1941 reached a level not seen since 1907. The following table shows how unpredictable infectious disease can be:

Diphtheria admissions 1930/31 to 1939/40

Year	Admissions
1930/31	2633
1931/32	3181
1932/33	3244
1933/34	2780
1934/35	2386
1935/36	3555
1936/37	2168
1937/38	1106
1938/39	888
1939/40	761

There can be no doubt that immunising children against diphtheria played a significant part in reducing the level of diphtheria in the community. Scarlet fever, measles, rubella and mumps reached epidemic proportions during 1939/40, but the only really notable development to emerge from these epidemics was that sulphapyridine was found to bring excellent results as a treatment for measles patients suffering from bronchopneumonia. In terms of the world-wide struggle to combat infectious disease, 1940 was a notable year. Australian scientist Howard Florey, whilst at Oxford, managed to develop penicillin—first discovered by Scottish scientist Alexander Fleming —for medical use. Given the huge numbers of Allied military personnel being injured in the fighting or suffering from war-related illnesses, Florey's break-through could hardly have been more timely. In terms of treatment patterns, in the days before effective chemical treatments of infectious diseases, it was often difficult for medical staff to determine when it was safe to return a patient to the community. In the late 1930s and early 1940s the hospital was slowly moving towards initiating shorter-term stays.

The only major construction work undertaken at the hospital during 1939/40 was the rebuilding of the ambulance station and quarters, garages and workshops. Given the wartime shortages of labour and materials and finance, it was recognised that the program of expansion and improvements which Scholes had been urging was unlikely to be brought to fruition. The annual report, however, recorded that one potentially serious problem had been successfully tackled by good management:

> Long before the outbreak of war, steps had been taken to lay in stocks of drugs, sera, and equipment which are not produced locally. These stocks were drawn upon in the months preceding the declaration of war, but before this occurred they were replenished, and since that time opportunities have been taken of acquiring important goods at favourable prices, which are now not procurable. In this connection, the close and sagacious attention of the Dispenser, Mr. Thomas, has been of great value.

In 1940 many of Australia's young men were already facing great dangers in the armed services in defence of the nation, and many nurses were taking the same risks in a non-combative capacity. At a time of 'Blood and Iron', when courage, tenacity and moral fortitude were in such urgent demand and heroism was in the air, we recognise the dangers that the staff—particularly nursing and medical staff—at the hospital faced on a daily basis. Sandland, in his evocative paper on the history of the hospital, presents the remarkable but not altogether atypical story of one young trainee nurse's experiences, and some intriguing glimpses of the day-to-day running of the hospital:

> In 1940 a 19 year old nurse came here on rotation for the first six months of her third year training, the first having been spent at the Austin, her parent hospital, and the second at the Queen Victoria hospital. She arrived to find soldiers everywhere, also some prisoners of war with Amoebic Dysentery. She was set to

work in a Scarlet Fever ward, and in the first couple of days there took pity on a crying child, picking him up. She was rostered off for the weekend, but by Sunday had a searingly sore throat. The next seven weeks were spent as an in-patient with Scarlet Fever and some of its complications. At first she found some relief from the extreme pain in the regular throat douches, but then had to grapple subsequently with bilateral suppurating middle ear infection, acute Rheumatism and finally Nephritis.

She was then put back on duty as a nightnurse (one of two for a ward with 40 children with Whooping Cough). She developed sinusitis, necessitating further time off, then worked as an attending nurse for our motorised ambulance service, three or four diphtheria cases being collected each trip, from as far away as Moorabbin.

Because of time lost through illness, she spent ten months at Fairfield instead of six, working a 52-hour week for a weekly wage of 27 shillings. (Twenty years earlier Scholes had pleaded with the Board to pay probationer nurses £52 a year, and in the end they had agreed.) When the nurse returned to the Austin Hospital to complete her training, she was found to have tuberculous infection of lymph nodes in the neck. Six of her classmates developed pulmonary tuberculosis. Sandland commented:

> Yes, nursing at this time had real hazards, and when it was announced that you worked at Fairfield hospital there tended to be social ostracism as well. Hence it's all the more amazing that 19 year old nurse eventually chose to return as a permanent member of our nursing teaching staff.[7]

It would be possible to give the name of this brave young woman but it seems fitting that, like the Unknown Soldier of World War I, she remains nameless and her story is allowed to stand in honour of the many thousands of nurses and other medical and para-medical staff who have invested their energy, skill and courage in the hospital and the community over the years.

The year 1940/41 saw the highest number of admissions in the history of the hospital. With 7435 admissions—859 higher than the previous year—the hospital had was exceptionally busy. The number of naval, military and air force patients admitted was 1345, compared with 1410 for the preceding twelve months. Most of these cases occurred during the six months to December 1940, and nearly all were mumps, rubella or tonsillitis. The demand for beds decreased as the epidemics of these diseases waned, and also with the establishment of military hospitals. From March to July 1941, admissions consisted mainly of comparatively few cases of scarlet fever, diphtheria and meningitis.

The number of civilian cases (6090) was high, exceeding by 143 the previous highest number in 1931/32. Scarlet fever and diphtheria accounted

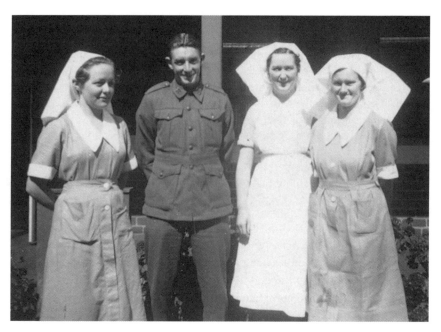

A returned soldier at Fairfield for rehabilitation, 1944.

for 4621, or about three-quarters of these. In 1940/41, 127 people died, 102 of these being young children—62 with whooping cough and 41 with diphtheria. Describing these events, Scholes noted:

> The epidemic of scarlet fever, which began in the spring of 1938, continued . . . and at the time of writing [October 1941] shows no real signs of abating . . . Only eight deaths occurred among the scarlet fever patients. Nowadays we can relieve quickly the most violent toxic manifestations by means of anti-toxin; that is to say, very few patients should, and very few do, die of toxaemia. We can treat successfully all the local and general septic infections of scarlet fever; that is to say, few should die of sepsis or pyaemia. In short, few patients should die of scarlet fever, from any cause whatever, in the actual course of that disease . . . On some occasions during the year it became necessary to restrict admission of patients to scarlet fever wards. All wards available for this disease were continuously occupied, and at times when numbers went far beyond a safe limit, or when over-crowding persisted for an unduly long time, admission was restricted to patients dangerously ill, destitute, or without reasonable facilities at home. Such periods of restriction varied from two to six weeks.

The number of diphtheria patients admitted in 1935/36 had been 3555, and during 1939/40 only 761. Admissions were low for the first few months of 1941, but in January the seasonal rise began, which had been the usual feature of diphtheria in Melbourne for many years. In November there was a

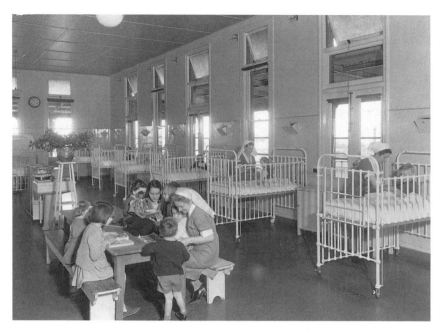

Convalescent children in the scarlet fever ward.

localised but very severe outbreak in an eastern suburb, due to *C. diphtheria intermedius*, the type of diphtheria bacillus responsible for the great epidemic of 1936. Scattered cases of infection due to this type gradually appeared over the city, and by March it was epidemic. Scholes commented:

> *C. Diphtheria gravis* now appeared as the dominant type, and the period March–June was characterised by a high proportion of malignant and very severe cases. It is pleasing that only 41 deaths occurred during the whole period [from 1498 diphtheria admissions]. Never in my experience has the efficacy of modern treatment of malignant diphtheria been made so manifest. So severe was the character of the disease that a large number of patients were admitted on the first day of illness.
>
> Partly as a result of this short but severe epidemic, an impetus was given to the practice of artificial immunization, which it is to be hoped will be sustained . . . I do not look for the best results [of the immunization campaign] till the majority of children are immunized in infancy, and tested, and if necessary re-immunized, when they enter school.

The impact of the war not only greatly increased admissions to the hospital but also placed pressure on staffing. The annual report for 1940/41 noted that 'Enlistments and home service needs made it necessary to conduct general activities with a group of employees much above the customary average age'. The pressure on hospital beds did, however, lead to ministerial approval being granted for the building of an additional wing to the nurses' home, and a new isolation wards block. It was not certain when these building projects would be started, but the hospital hoped that despite shortages of labour and material, building would 'proceed in the near future'.

The Commission of Public Health, having recognised that no provision existed for the isolation and treatment of patients suffering from diseases not indigenous to Australia, asked in March 1942 for the Board's approval for the establishment of a small Exotic Diseases Unit, to be built to the south of the hospital buildings. With so many Australian soldiers on active service overseas and liable to contact with all sorts of 'exotic' diseases, the erection of such a unit was urgent. The Board agreed, and the Department of Public Works began work on the site in November 1942; it was still not completed in 1944. The decision to establish this new unit was one of the few positive features of the war years, as the hospital struggled to maintain standards while coping with labour and material shortages, rationing and air raid precautions (the hospital's 5000 windows and fanlights all had to be fitted to meet lighting restrictions and given anti-scatter treatment). Plans which had been developed for improving and expanding hospital facilities had, in the main, to be placed on hold for the duration of the war.

The infectious disease pattern during 1941/42 was a somewhat unusual one. The scarlet fever epidemic which had been raging since the spring of 1938 began to decline in intensity in October 1941. At its peak between July and September the hospital had been under such pressure that it was unable to admit many of the patients presenting with scarlet fever. Although the epidemic was in decline after October, scarlet fever admissions remained high, ranging from 120 to 220 per month, but the hospital was now able to admit all scarlet fever cases. A short but severe diphtheria epidemic began in March 1941 but was over by July. This sudden rise in diphtheria infections puzzled medical staff as the disease had been 'very quiet' for three years and relapsed into this pattern after the March to July outbreak. Measles and whooping cough epidemics struck Melbourne in June. Though admissions in 1941/42 were down by 2734 on the previous year (from 7435 to 4701), staffing levels remained a serious problem for much of the year, the shortage of senior nurses being particularly severe.

The first nurse graduation ceremony to be held in Australia took place at the hospital in January 1943, when the first general nurses trained there received their certificates, Florence Nightingale Pledges, and the hospital badge. The Nightingale Pledge went as follows:

> I solemnly pledge myself before God and this Assembly to pass my life in purity and in the practice of my profession faithfully. I will abstain from what is deleterious and mischievous and will not take or knowingly administer any harm-

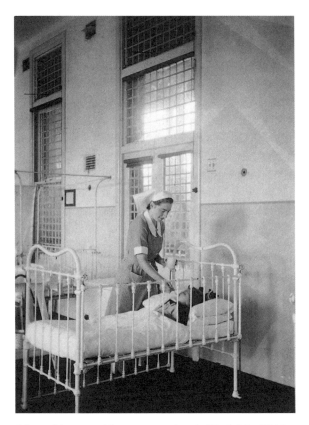

Nurse Adamson with a young patient in Ward 6 in 1944;
fear of wartime attack is evident in the strapping strips on
the windows, to prevent shatter.

ful drug. I will do all in my power to elevate the standard of my profession and will hold in confidence all private matters that come to my knowledge in the practice of my calling. With loyalty I will endeavour to aid the physician in his work and devote myself to those committed to my care.[8]

The Nightingale Pledge is essentially a shortened version of the Hippocratic Oath, the actual wording of which is not commonly known. A recent translation of the Hippocratic Oath reads as follows:

I will look upon him who shall have taught me this Art even as one of my parents. I will share my substance with him, and will supply his necessities, if he be in need. I will regard his offspring even as my own brethren, and I will teach them this Art, if they would learn it, without fee or covenant. I will impart this Art by precept, by lecture and by every mode of teaching, not only to my own sons but to the sons of him who has taught me, and to disciples bound by covenant and oath, according to the Law of Medicine.

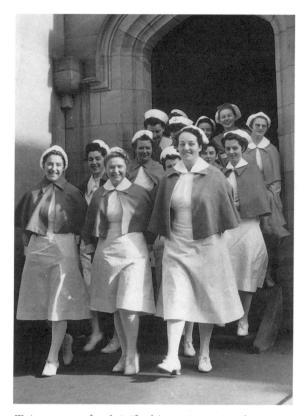

*Trainee nurses after their 'finals' examinations at the
University of Melbourne in 1944.*

The regimen I adopt shall be for the benefit of my patients according to my
ability and judgement, and not for their hurt or for any wrong. I will give no
deadly drug to any, though it be asked of me, nor will I counsel such, and
especially I will not aid a woman to procure abortion. Whatsoever house I enter,
there will I go for the benefit of the sick, refraining from all wrongdoing or cor-
ruption, and especially from the act of seduction, of male or female, or bond or
free. Whatsoever things I see or hear concerning the life of men, in my attendance on the sick or even apart therefrom, which ought not to be noised
abroad, I will keep silence thereon, counting such things to be as sacred secrets.[92]

A significant increase in nursing payments in January 1943 was the result
of a new award. The hospital was deprived of the services of Matron Burbidge
for four months in 1943, as the Director-General of Manpower asked her to

establish and organise the Nursing Control Division in Victoria. Despite the difficulties and demands related to the hostilities, the hospital managed to make some improvements to its facilities. Even in the dark days of 1943, a new X-ray plant and an operating theatre were put into operation through converting pre-existing buildings. The prevalence of scarlet fever continued during 1942/43 and was particularly severe during the last quarter of the year. The diphtheria admission rate was at its lowest since 1909, with admissions running at less than a quarter of the rate which had prevailed in the twenty years prior to the start of the decline in 1937.

A major typhoid (enteric) fever epidemic broke out in Melbourne in March 1943. Described as a 'classical "milk epidemic"' the outbreak started in Cheltenham, a bayside suburb some 13 miles from the centre of Melbourne. The origin of the outbreak was traced to a carrier at a dairy farm from which one of the area's milk distributors obtained his supplies. The contagion caused 436 cases, of whom 23 died. Due to the prevalence of scarlet fever and problems caused by understaffing, the hospital treated only 114 (7 fatalities) of these patients. Scholes was a member of a Consultative Advisory Committee established by the government to tackle the emergency, and helped arrange the opening of wards for typhoid patients at several Melbourne hospitals.

Typhoid fever is an acute infectious disease of the digestive tract, caused by the bacterium *Salmonella typhi*. The disease is usually contracted through contaminated food or water and symptoms include fever, cough, headache, diarrhoea or constipation and rash. It is an ancient disease that can be recognised back to the time of Hippocrates. It was clearly differentiated from other fevers in the 1820s and given the name *fievre typhoide* in France in 1829. Typhoid was introduced to Australia on various immigrant and convict ships. Large outbreaks occurred after the discovery of gold in 1851, and severe epidemics occurred in Aboriginal settlements, with many deaths. Typhoid was a major killer in early Melbourne, increasing markedly in the 1880s. Largely as a result of a 'clean-up' campaign pushing for improved sanitation, typhoid deaths fell dramatically in the 1890s. There is now an effective vaccine which protects against both typhoid and the related (though milder) paratyphoid fever.

Whooping cough and measles were almost totally absent from Melbourne during 1943/44, and Dr Scholes himself described the year as 'a singularly uneventful one'—which was good news for the people of Melbourne. Scarlet fever admissions, however, reached 3506, which was then the highest in the history of the hospital. The incidence of diphtheria continued to fall with only 544 admissions—the lowest for thirty-five years. Penicillin was used to treat a variety of cases during the year, but with disappointing results.

In December 1943 the *Ministry of Health Act* was passed by Parliament, and became operative on 1 July 1944. Under the terms of the Act all health matters and all state medical services were brought under one control and the Department of Health was made responsible for administering all health-related legislation.

Victory Europe year, 1945, saw work begin on a new boiler house, improvements to the nurses' home and a new three-storey isolation block, an important addition to the hospital. It was known as the Scholes' Block in recognition of the Medical Superintendent's long association with the hospital. Two new appointments in 1945, of a personnel officer and a welfare officer, pointed to the growing awareness of staff needs and the competition among hospitals to recruit high quality staff:

> [in an] effort to help towards nurse recruitment and the maintenance of the pleasant atmosphere for which the Board had always striven, a new appointment was made of a personnel officer, or social director, to the nursing staff, and also a welfare officer to the household staff, to assist in the adjustment of hospital household staff, particularly the many New Australians just then coming into the country.[10]

The epidemic of scarlet fever which had raged since early in 1938 finally came to end early in 1945. In June there were only 114 scarlet fever admissions, the lowest monthly number since 1938. Diphtheria, measles and whooping cough admissions also remained low. Only 4686 patients were admitted during the year and Scholes, writing in September 1945, noted that the 'autumn and winter have been the quietest since 1915'.

Dr F. M. (later Sir Macfarlane) Burnet was appointed Consultant Epidemiologist in 1946, and Dr E. V. Keogh was appointed Consultant Bacteriologist. The fact that medical scientists of international stature were keen to be associated with the hospital reflects the growing reputation it was building as an important centre for research into infectious diseases. Another sign of growing maturity and progressive attitude was the visit of Matron Burbidge to America in 1946. Burbidge (who had been elected as a nursing representative to the Nurses' Board of Victoria during the war) had been appointed

Australian delegate to the Florence Nightingale Foundation Grand Council and the International Congress of Nurses. The hospital had really come of age, and was known and respected not only within Australia but also in the international medical community.

The trend towards lower rates of admission continued during 1945/46 (3479 admissions). Scholes noted that 'A number of infectious diseases were moderately prevalent, but there were no great epidemics, and generally these prevalences affected a particular part of the metropolitan area, and failed to become general. I do not remember a year in which this tendency was so pronounced.' The admission rates for both scarlet fever and diphtheria continued to fall, but an outbreak of poliomyelitis, during which 243 patients were admitted, darkened what would otherwise have been a relatively benign period for infectious diseases. Scholes presented a detailed description and analysis of the poliomyelitis epidemic in the 1945/46 annual report:

> Spread had occurred geographically along the main railways and highways from New South Wales. From July to October scattered cases occurred over the whole metropolitan area, but every focus in the thickly populated areas died out without any notable incidence of clinical cases. From October to March the vast majority of all cases came from the Eastern and North-Eastern suburbs, adjacent outlying areas, and country districts. So far as the metropolitan area was concerned, the epidemic was obviously over by the end of February. Thus once again poliomyelitis in Melbourne has been proved *not* to be essentially a disease of the late summer and autumn months. Once again it has taken about eight months to run its course, irrespective of the season of the year.

Scholes commented on some unusual features of the epidemic:

1. As stated, although one or more cases occurred in each thickly populated municipality, the total number of cases for all industrial and working-class residential areas was very small. Yet a large susceptible child population could be assumed, for practically no cases had occurred since the 1937 epidemic.
2. Of the 243 patients, 79 were over 15 years of age, and only 47 under five years of age. The term infantile paralysis appears to be a misnomer. Only three patients were infants. Adults suffered much more severely from paralysis, and seven of the nine deaths were of patients more than fifteen years old.
3. There was the usual preponderance of males, both as regards to incidence and fatality.
4. There were no fewer than seven instances of familial incidence. All of these patients exhibited paralysis . . . Such a large number of familial cases is very unusual.

    Respirator treatment was necessary in 21 cases, but in some of the patients the outlook was hopeless from the beginning. In three fatal cases respirator treatment was not applied. In four cases of respiratory paralysis, respirator treatment was not necessary. Of the twenty-one patients, six died, three made good recovery, three made fairly good recovery, with limited residual paralysis, and in nine extensive residual paralysis of body and limbs persisted ...

Most of the adult polio patients were badly paralysed, and it was necessary to provide after-care for them in hospital. The hospital appointed one full-time physiotherapist (later this was increased to four). Some patients were eventually transferred to other hospitals or their homes for after-care, but on 30 June, 21 still remained at the hospital.

A consultative council was set up by the government to make plans for accommodation and care of present and future polio patients throughout the state. Attention was given to the difficulty of providing for adolescents and adults, where paralysis in many cases was likely to be extensive, prolonged or permanent. Scholes, perhaps wishing to get a few things off his chest as he approached retirement, also presented in his report a spirited plea for changes to the hospital's role and functions and, in particular, to the question of diseases admissible to the hospital:

> I have repeatedly (1931, 1937, 1938) referred to the need for recognition of the changing functions of fever hospitals, and for the more intelligent use of such hospitals. The two original functions still stand, and are:–
> 1. The accommodation and treatment of all patients suffering from infectious disease, who cannot be attended to efficiently and safely in their homes or in other hospitals.
> 2. The separation from the general community of such persons who are a danger to others.
>
> The relative importance of these two function is constantly changing, according to the behaviour of various infectious diseases and additions to scientific knowledge. It is no longer rational to deny the benefits of hospital treatment to serious and necessitous cases of infectious pharyngitis, laryngitis and pneumonia. Tens of thousands of such patients have been admitted and treated in this hospital during the past generation, having been sent in as possibly suffering from diphtheria or other admissible disease ... I recommend that the suggestion be made to the Minister that the following diseases be added to the list of those which may be treated in this hospital:–
>
> Acute Infective Pharyngitis.
> Pneumonia and Bronchopneumonia.
> Puerperal Fever.
>
> For the past thirty years complicated, severe, and necessitous cases of Mumps, Varicella, and Rubella have been admitted and treated in hospital, and it is also suggested that these be included.

Scholes' words suggest that the hospital had a long-term policy of admitting anyone whom it considered appropriate, regardless of the 'admissible diseases' list, and that alterations to the official list would simply recognise hospital practice. His strongly worded recommendations were heeded, for he was able to record in the 1947 annual report that all of his recommendations regarding additions to the hospital's admissible diseases list had been accepted.

The final period to be considered in this chapter, 1946/47, saw the lowest number of admissions since 1925/26 (2964). This was brought about largely by the fact that scarlet fever admissions were the lowest since 1937/38 (1136) and diphtheria admissions the lowest since 1906/07 (233). While there were still a few poliomyelitis cases appearing—with the fear of a major outbreak causing continuing concern—measles, whooping cough and other common infectious diseases all led to only moderate levels of admission. While this was, of course, good news, it did mean that 'from an economic point of view, the hospital was in an unsound position' as a result of having such a large proportion of vacant beds.

The immediate post-war years was a time of change and development for the hospital during which important discussions were initiated with the government regarding legislative changes to enable the hospital to treat general medical and surgical patients. This change would not only fill the empty beds brought about by the decline of infectious disease rates, but also encourage more nurses to train at the hospital and thus help to resolve staffing problems. The hospital was also giving some thought to the advantages of 'affiliation of some kind with a large teaching hospital', and planning to expand the scope and scale of its research activities. In 1947 the hospital was on the threshold of important and far-reaching changes. This was also the last year that the hospital would use the name Queen's Memorial Infectious Diseases Hospital; henceforth it would be known as Fairfield Hospital.

Fairfield Hospital
1948–1969

Fairfield is in good heart.

Fairfield Hospital Annual Report, 1966.

I doubt if there are many hospitals in the world where such a variety of interesting medical conditions can be seen and studied as are being admitted to Fairfield. Positions as Resident Medical Officers at the hospital are eagerly sought after, as it is recognised that this experience cannot be gained at any other hospital, and provides a valuable experience for future practice.

Fairfield Hospital Annual Report, 1955.

In the 1950s, Fairfield Hospital was a large institution (600 beds plus and sited on an area of over 20 acres), but most of the buildings were old and in need of renovation or replacement. At that time, the future of the hospital was then in doubt because it was widely believed that infectious diseases had been largely conquered. This false optimism had been engendered by a number of factors: diphtheria had been virtually eliminated by immunisation; polio virus had been isolated and effective vaccines to combat this dreaded disease were soon to be available; a rapidly expanding armamentarium of antibiotics was evolving which would enable nearly all bacterial diseases to be treated successfully. The number of patients being admitted to Fairfield Hospital had been falling and, because of similar trends, infectious diseases hospitals were being progressively closed in many parts of the developed world. It was, therefore, not surprising that those in control of capital grants to hospitals were not imbued with any sense of urgency to rebuild Fairfield Hospital. It was to be the mid-1960s before the hospital reasserted itself as a leading Australian and World Centre for Communicable Diseases. The survival of Fairfield Hospital during this period of uncertainty was a tribute to the determination of successive Boards of Management and to strong medical and administrative leadership.

Fairfield Hospital Annual Report, 1979.

THE HOSPITAL'S 1948 annual report was entitled 'Fairfield Hospital'. Unofficially this name had been used almost since its inception, but this was the first official recognition. Due to lack of documentation it is not possible to ascertain if this alteration had been either instituted or agreed to by the state government. It was to be 27 October 1954 before the Legislative

Assembly passed 'A Bill Relating to Infectious Diseases Hospitals', legally sanctioning the change of name. The Bill in fact seems to leave the hospital's name optional—'The Queen's Memorial Infectious Diseases Hospital at Fairfield shall be a hospital for the care and treatment of persons suffering from infectious disease and may be called the "Fairfield Hospital" '. Of more note than the change in the hospital's nomenclature was the resignation of the Medical Superintendent, Dr F. V. Scholes CMG, MD, BSc (Melb), DPh (Cantab), FRCAP, on 1 April 1948. Scholes had given forty years of service to the hospital—an amazing thirty-eight of which were as Medical Superintendent. A study of the hospital published a few years later contained the following well-deserved tribute to him:

> The reputation of Dr Scholes as a world authority on infectious disease is well known. The names of Scholes and Fairfield became synonymous, and through his textbooks he gained a worldwide reputation. As a teacher he was naturally gifted and his writings and teachings have been quoted in many parts of the world. Fairfield will greatly miss such a personality.[1]

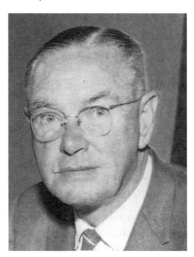

Dr H. McLorinan, who had been Deputy Medical Superintendent for many years and who had outstanding qualifications and experience in infectious disease, was appointed Medical Superintendent. Another important development was the appointment of Dr A. A. Ferris as bacteriologist. Ferris had extensive experience with the Australian Army Medical Corps during World War II, and prior to his appointment to Fairfield had been Assistant Director of the Public Health Laboratory in Melbourne.

In many ways 1948 was a watershed year for the hospital: not only did its name and senior officer change, but legislation was enacted which enabled it

Dr H. McLorinan, Medical Superintendent 1948–60.

to treat general medical and surgical patients. It was hoped that this would solve the perennial problem of recruiting sufficient nurses. Despite employing a special recruitment officer (Sister V. Houghton) and preparing and distributing an 'attractive brochure' highlighting the joys of working at the hospital, the problem remained so acute that the hospital admitted in its 1948 annual report that 'Owing to staff shortages it was again not found practicable to admit all types of diseases gazetted as admissible to the hospital'.

In attempting to resolve the shortage of nursing staff the hospital broke with tradition and entered into a radical and ambitious relationship with the Royal Melbourne Hospital. A section of the 1948 annual report entitled 'Future Development of the Hospital' described the changes:

> For the past few years two factors have caused concern to the Board of Management. Firstly, it was realised that from an economic point of view the larger proportion of empty beds in the hospital was unsound. Secondly, that the continued shortage of nurses placed the hospital in a position in which it would be quite unable to cope with an epidemic of any size.
>
> On ascertaining that the Royal Melbourne hospital was anxious to institute a wider general training for their nurses, negotiations were begun between the two hospitals in an endeavour to arrange a combined system of nurse training for both hospitals.
>
> As a preliminary step four wards of twenty-six beds each have been opened at Fairfield for sub-acute medical and surgical cases. These patients are transferred from the Royal Melbourne hospital on the understanding that they are the type which can be easily evacuated in time of epidemic emergency. These wards are staffed by Fairfield sisters and Royal Melbourne hospital trainees. At the time of writing the wards are functioning smoothly. In addition to supplying a further thirty nurses to the Fairfield staff, available for an emergency, the net result is an increase of 104 beds to Melbourne's acute hospital bed position.

Thus on 1 July a 'General Division'—four wards accommodating 104 sub-acute and convalescent medical and surgical patients—opened at Fairfield. In its first year of operations the General Division admitted 1487 patients, all of whom were transferred from the Royal Melbourne Hospital. Dr McLorinan's first months in charge of the hospital were marked by notable developments. The opening of these general beds necessitated the hospital providing accommodation for thirty Royal Melbourne Hospital nurses and, although the structure and basic functions of the Board of Management remained the same, the hospital now had official contact with the Hospital Commission and the Health Department. By providing beds for general patients from the Royal Melbourne, Fairfield alleviated its shortage of nurses and freed beds at the Royal Melbourne for urgent general and surgical cases. It also reduced costs to the municipalities which contributed to Fairfield's operating costs. (The annual report for 1947/48 noted: 'The cost of treatment of patients in the General Section will, in no way, be the liability of the Contributory Councils').

Another interesting development in 1948 was the hospital's participation with the Walter and Eliza Hall Institute and female volunteer university students in testing the possibilities of the experimental transmission of rubella virus to human volunteers. Fairfield provided a ward block and diagnostic and clinical assistance. This involvement reflected the high priority that Dr McLorinan placed in the research component of the hospital. His strong recommendations won the approval of Board to increase the facilities for research into infectious diseases. In the 1949 annual report, Dr McLorinan explained his commitment to research:

> The position of the laboratory in modern hospital practice yearly assumes more importance. This is perhaps more especially true in a fever hospital, where accurate bacteriological diagnosis is necessary for a decision on the correct specific form of treatment. The volume of laboratory work has increased and will continue to increase, but the resulting close relation between clinician and laboratory worker has a further outcome. It brings to light those problems which might be overlooked by either alone—by the physician remaining at the bedside and by the Research worker in the splendid isolation of his laboratory.

Fairfield was now recognised as an 'Approved Research Institution' and employed research staff of the quality of Dr A. A. Ferris and Dr W. Stevenson. The experience and expertise of Fairfield staff was reinforced by the close liaison the hospital had developed with the Victorian Health Department and the Walter and Eliza Hall Institute of Medical Research. Overall it is fair to say that the hospital had managed—often against the odds—to establish an excellent research base. In the decades which followed the hospital's research arm would, as McLorinan foresaw, grow dramatically in scope, scale and importance.

Although the mutually beneficial arrangement with the Royal Melbourne hospital had a positive effect on Fairfield's nursing shortage, the problem was far from resolved, as the annual report for 1949 noted:

> The nursing shortage has caused acute anxiety throughout the year, and is not altogether due to the general shortage of labour. The increase in recent months of admissions of poliomyelitis cases placed a great strain and much additional work. Fortunately, the marked decrease in admissions of minor infectious cases enabled the polio cases to be adequately cared for, but in the event of a major epidemic of an infectious nature occurring the position would be extremely serious.
>
> If, as appears likely, the endeavour to establish a Training School does not materialise, some other means of attracting nurses must be found.
>
> The problem is continuously under consideration by both the Board, the Medical Superintendent, Matron and other executive officers, and is undoubtedly the most serious problem facing the hospital.

Fairfield devoted a lot of time and energy to its 'most serious problem'. It entered into negotiations with the Royal Melbourne Hospital for the two hospitals to jointly open a Nurses Training School at Fairfield, but this

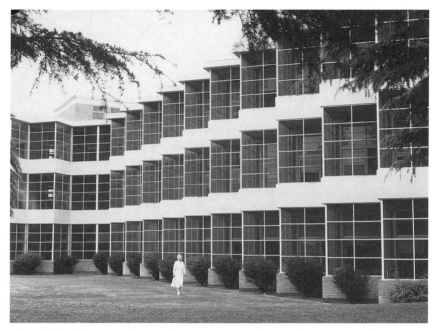

The Scholes Block, opened in April 1950, was named as a tribute to Dr Scholes. Matron Burbidge stands outside.

initiative came to nothing due to the Hospital Commission's plans to establish regional training schools for nurses.

There were a number of significant additions to the hospital in 1949, including a new isolation block, the F. V. Scholes Block (a substantial building comprising three floors, with single rooms and balconies), which was officially opened in April by the Minister for Health, C. P. Gartside. In a sporting gesture, three tennis courts were constructed in the hospital grounds—the Board's tribute to the staff for their work during the poliomyelitis epidemic. In a sign of the times, the extension of hospital activities and the increase in car ownership made it necessary 'to create a Car Park of some magnitude'.

This epidemic of poliomyelitis occurred towards the end of March 1949 and resulted in over 200 admissions to the hospital. McLorinan described it in the annual report:

> The change in character of this disease first noted in the big epidemic of 1937–38 is still in evidence this year. The age incidence has now shifted to the older children and young adults, with the dangerous bulbar and respiratory types more common in the older age groups. The mortality among adults particularly males over 20 years, has been rather heavy in the present outbreak, and

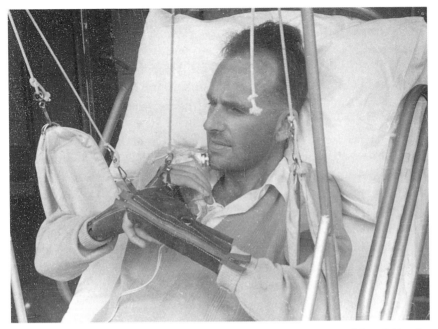

Keith Davis, photographed in Ward 14 in the early 1950s, was a victim of the 1949 polio epidemic. He is shaving, with specialised gloves and pulleys.

has been chiefly caused by the high incidence of pulmonary complications in the respirator cases.

In the purely 'bulbar' types with pharyngeal and laryngeal involvement, the efficient use of postural drainage, combined with tracheotomy, has given dramatic results in some cases.

The year 1948/49 also saw the formation of an auxiliary to assist in raising funds for the hospital, and to work for the well-being of the patients of the four general wards (because of the closed nature of the infectious disease wards the Auxiliary could not service these wards) by providing canteen and trolley services, and to give priceless voluntary service. The Auxiliary not only provided important services to the hospital community, but also helped to humanise, to give heart and warmth, to the whole hospital environment. The jubilee history of the hospital published in 1954—only a few years after the Auxiliary was formed—already described its work as of 'inestimable value to the hospital'.[2] In the decades to come many thousands of patients and staff who benefited either directly or indirectly from the selfless and unremitting work of the Auxiliary would have reason to echo these sentiments.

Other significant events that year included the election of the first female chair in the history of the hospital, when Cr Nellie Ibbott was elected on the retirement of Malcolm Parker; the resignation of Neep as secretary, with B. D. Dynon, FCIS, AASA, ACCA, FIHS, appointed to replace him. Matron Burbidge received a Rockefeller Foundation Fellowship—the first to a member of the Australian nursing profession—entitling her to a postgraduate course of study in Canada and the United States. During her absence, A. J. Mason, having been Deputy Matron for a number of years, acted in her stead. Fairhaven Women's Clinic was closed in July 1949; the government had proposed to convert it into a women's prison holding sixty prisoners but was later forced to back down in the face of public opposition. The government remained attracted to the idea of siting a prison in the area, and in June 1953 it was announced that a women's prison to be called Fairlea would be built near the south-western boundary of the hospital. The College of Nursing, Australia was founded (an important step in the professionalisation and representation of nursing and nurses), as was the Commonwealth Institute of Child Health.

In the 1948/49 report of his first full year in charge of the hospital, McLorinan brought high intelligence and decades of experience in treating infectious diseases to his reflections on 'The Future of Fever Hospitals'. His comments on the declining incidence of some of the most common infectious diseases are the future of fever hospitals are worth quoting at length:

> In the decade preceding World War II the major proportion of fever hospital beds was occupied by diphtheria and scarlet fever patients. The influence of immunisation in reducing the influence of diphtheria must now be accepted as an established fact. The decline in the morbidity of scarlet fever, however, is more difficult to explain, and one hesitates to advance the suggestion that the constant war being waged on streptococcal organisms by the mass use of sulphonamides and penicillin is at last having an effect.
>
> The result of the lessened incidence of these two diseases has been to free a large number of beds in fever hospitals for other uses. The problem of how best to use these empty beds has been one that has occupied the minds of hospital authorities. In many cases the fever hospital has lost its identity as such, and has become a general hospital or attached to a general hospital. It seems a pity that such should be the case when it is remembered that a great deal of the work in preventive medicine which has largely brought about this radical change, has emanated from the fever hospitals themselves. The specialised nature of their work has always made them the centres of teaching and research in certain aspects of public health and preventive medicine.
>
> It seems logical, therefore, to suggest that the future extension of fever hospitals should be along lines which would enable them to continue and enlarge this aspect of their work. A number of diseases of bacterial or virus origin, not

necessarily infectious, at present treated in general hospitals could be admitted to fever hospitals. The admission of these diseases to fever hospitals would not only relieve the acute bed shortage in the general hospitals, but would enable them to continue as specialised units dealing with the treatment and prevention of disease and acting as centres for teaching and research, especially in matters pertaining to public health and epidemiology.

McLorinan stated that the Board intended to place an increased emphasis on research, and expressed the hope that association with the Walter and Eliza Hall Institute and the Commonwealth Serum Laboratories would enable further valuable research work in both bacterial and virus diseases.

Fairfield had experienced a dramatic, indeed precipitous, decline in admissions due to the decreasing incidence of infectious diseases. It is clear that he was in effect mounting a bold, persuasively argued campaign to reposition the hospital by extending the scope of its functions. While there can be no doubt of McLorinan's commitment to research and his personal capacity for flexible and creative responses to medical and administrative challenges, we can also read between the lines to see a man with a deep and longstanding commitment and loyalty to a hospital which appeared to be moving towards obsolescence—a victim of changing times rather than any inherent weaknesses or failures. Clearly, as the decade drew to an end, the future of the hospital—not for the first time—was looking precarious.

The pattern of reduced demand for specialised infectious disease beds at Fairfield continued into the 1950s. By 1956 the relationship that Fairfield had developed with the Royal Melbourne was extended and Fairfield took over the short-term management of patients suffering from chronic disease. By the end of the decade Fairfield had entered into negotiations with the Royal Children's Hospital regarding the possibility of admitting children for surgery at Fairfield from the Royal Children's surgery waiting list. The policy of lending beds and facilities to other hospitals was continued throughout the 1950s; it was the early 1960s before the rate of infectious diseases accelerated and demand for specialised infectious disease beds at Fairfield increased.

The year 1948/49 also saw the reorganisation of the hospital's laboratory services and the formation of the Fairfield Epidemiological Research Unit, which opened in February. The opening of this unit was made possible by a substantial grant from the National Health and Medical Research Council and the co-operation of the Victorian Health Department and the Walter and Eliza Hall Institute. In keeping with McLorinan's policy of building up the hospital's research function, the 'old' laboratory was refitted as the virus department of the Epidemiological Research Unit. Work at this small laboratory was led by Dr Frank Burnet, who used the laboratory to provide a clinical focus for his studies in virology. Burnet has been described as 'founding patron' of Fairfield's Research Centre.[3]

The first year of the new decade also saw Fairfield's Exotic Diseases Unit admit its first Hansen's disease (leprosy) patients. Although the number of Hansen's disease patients treated remained relatively small, this historically notorious disease was to become a significant area of special interest for the hospital.

Matron Burbidge, recently returned from her successful Rockefeller Foundation Fellowship, presented a report on the hospital in the 1950 annual report. It reflected the major preoccupation of the hospital in that it concentrated on the shortage of nursing staff:

> The problem of the provision of nursing staff for hospitals is today urgent in any hospital. In any epidemic hospital where the number of patients fluctuates greatly, the problem is even greater. In the past, during an epidemic, when no labour shortage existed, it was possible to meet increased needs for nursing staff by the temporary appointment of trained nurses and of untrained nurse assistants. For the last ten years the grave labour shortage has made this a plan impossible to implement, thus leaving the Community, served by Fairfield hospital, with the ever-present risk of an epidemic with which the hospital could not cope. From time to time, some cases of Infectious Diseases have been unable to secure admission owing to staff shortage, and all the time there have been beds lying empty in fully equipped wards, at a time when Melbourne is so urgently needing hospital beds.

The poliomyelitis epidemic which started in March 1949 continued to rage in 1950 and became 'the second largest poliomyelitis epidemic in the history of the state'. In 1949/50 Fairfield admitted 492 patients, 35 of whom died.

In describing this epidemic, McLorinan noted that while in extent and severity it was not comparable to the 'great Victorian Epidemic of 1937–1938', it did present some unusual features. He drew attention to three factors which differentiated it from previous epidemics. The tendency for the disease to affect older age groups than previous epidemics, and the higher death rate and more severe crippling among older victims, led McLorinan to suggest that the widespread name 'infantile paralysis' was no longer appropriate. He also noted that an 'accumulation of evidence' suggested an association between combined diphtheria and whooping cough injections, and paralytic poliomyelitis. Concerns about the alleged dangers of inoculations would, over the following decades, undermine efforts to achieve universal protection from a number of common infectious diseases—whooping cough being a prime example. McLorinan also noted a statistically significant over-representation of pregnant women among the victims—16 of the 34 women over the age of

Hansen's disease (leprosy) has been a source of horror and distress to people for centuries. This disabling and deforming disease was mentioned in Egyptian papyri over four thousand years ago, and makes frequent appearances in the Bible. It appears in sources from ancient Mesopotamia, India, China and Japan, but it is possible that other skin diseases may have been mistaken for leprosy. The first mention in England is in 638 CE. It was prevalent in Europe in the middle ages, and special hospitals, lazar-houses or lazarettos were built for the sufferers. As there was no known cure, people stayed in the lazar-houses for life. In 1318 the King of France, Philip V, proposed that all lepers should be burned alive. A less horrifying but still unpleasant treatment was the application of a mixture of adders boiled with leeks. Although all treatments were ineffective, leprosy disappeared from Italy in the sixteenth century, and from France, England and Germany in the following century. The high mortality caused by the Black Death may have been partly responsible for the decline of leprosy, as foci of the disease were wiped out.

Leprosy may have been brought to Australia by Chinese and Indian migrants in the nineteenth century, or by the crews of pearling luggers. In the 1867 *Report on Leprosy* by the Royal College of Physicians, only Victoria reported any definite incidence of the disease— among Chinese on the goldfields. In the other Australian colonies the disease had perhaps simply not been diagnosed.

Leprosy is caused by the bacillus *Mycobacterium leprae*, first described by Hansen in 1874. Destruction of the peripheral nerves leads to a loss of sensation which, together with tissue degeneration, may result in the extremities becoming deformed and eroded. It is transmitted directly from person to person, and can be discharged in large quantities from the nose or sores of an infected person. However, Hansen's disease is not particularly contagious and long or repeated contact is usually necessary. Accidental transmission by improperly sterilised hypodermic and tattoo needles has occurred.

twenty were pregnant on admission. Fairfield doctor, Frank Foster, had considerable experience and expertise at vaginal delivery of the babies of polio victims. This was safer than caesarean delivery, but very difficult.

Attempting to summarise the 'Lessons of the Epidemic' in the 1950 annual report, McLorinan readily admitted that the significance of his observations on the epidemic were 'not easy to assess', but nonetheless provided positive research opportunities:

> The factors of muscle fatigue, injections into a limb, tonsillectomy and pregnancy all appear to render muscles, or their corresponding motor nerve cells, more susceptible to the paralytic effect of the poliomyelitis virus. For the present it is sufficient to say that they provide a line of research into the pathogenesis of paralytic poliomyelitis. The recently formed epidemiological research unit at Fairfield has already commenced work on virus infections of the central nervous system; but further investigations are dependent on an adequate supply of monkeys, the only laboratory animal which is susceptible to poliomyelitis.

As Medical Superintendent, McLorinan took every opportunity to explain the changing role of the hospital and specifically to promote his vision of Fairfield as centre for research into infectious diseases. In the 1950 annual report he presented a section entitled 'Modern Antibiotic Drugs: Their Effect on Fever Hospitals, and Hospital Statistics'. He attempted to explain how modern antibiotics had considerably reduced the average period of hospital admissions and this in turn had caused the hospital's statistics to show a lower daily average of occupied beds—statistics which, if read simplistically and unsympathetically, could give a fallacious impression of the calibre of the hospital. Similarly, he argued that the relatively high cost per bed of a hospital like Fairfield was inherent in its specialised role and functions:

> A similar fallacy is seen in the compilation of a figure representing the cost per bed. An efficient teaching hospital must always be at a disadvantage in this respect. In the first place a progressive hospital should be in the forefront in clinical trials and research, expensive items involving the purchase and clinical trial of drugs which preliminary tests have shown to be worthy of such a trial. Many of these drugs may prove to be disappointing and may be subsequently discarded. Others may prove to be valuable curative weapons and have capabilities undreamt of by the laboratory discoverer, until tested by the clinician. Teaching hospitals invariably purchase these drugs in the early stages of their production when their cost is usually prohibitive to the ordinary patient. Clinical trials, along with laboratory control in the hospital prove their worth, the drug is produced in quantity and the price drops steeply. Whatever the result, however, the cost of the drug at its initial stage of production is added to the cost per bed of the progressive hospital, while the cost per bed of the hospital which is content to wait until the drug has proved itself remains low.
> Fairfield as a special university teaching hospital owes a duty to the community to give a lead in matters affecting the management of communicable diseases, as well as carrying out clinical and laboratory research. The superficial effect of this policy may be seen in an increase in the cost per bed and a low daily average. In the long range view, however, the community must reap the benefit.

No doubt under McLorinan's guidance, the Board of Management decided in 1951 to adopt a 'new policy' for the hospital. In the annual report it explained the move thus:

> The progress made in preventive methods in connection with infectious diseases continued with the discovery of more potent and effective drugs, and has had the dual result of fewer admissions to and quicker discharges from hospital. For example, scarlet fever treatment has reduced hospitalisation from an approximate average of four weeks to one of ten days. Early in the year, the Board reconsidered hospital policy with the two-fold object of giving greater community service and reducing infectious treatment costs. In planning its new policy the Board proceeded on the basis that the paramount considerations were—
> (a) the treatment and isolation of infectious diseases,
> (b) the necessity of being ready in all respects to cope with a major epidemic at short notice,
> (c) the training of nurses and medical students in the care and treatment of infectious diseases, and
> (d) research in all phases of preventive medicine and in the treatment of infectious diseases.

In the same report the Board also noted that a survey of the hospital's operations had shown that after providing for the 'normal' intake of infectious disease patients, up to 230 beds could be made available for short-term non-infectious cases—patients who could be quickly discharged or transferred if the hospital faced a severe epidemic and suddenly needed their beds.

The continuing shortage of nursing staff remained critical, but it was hoped that the new Melbourne School of Nursing—originally planned by Fairfield and Royal Melbourne hospitals—which came into operation in 1951 would go a long way to resolving this problem. This development in nursing education was described as a 'milestone' in the history of the hospital.[4] Under this scheme, trainee nurses now came to Fairfield for part of their training, and passed on to the Royal Melbourne, the Women's and Queen Victoria hospitals in turn. As well as the new training scheme, the Board at this time decided to introduce a scheme to 'enlist trained nurses from England [clearly they meant Britain and Ireland] and certain Continental countries'. The combination of the new School of Nursing and the policy of 'importing' trained nurses meant that the Board had to push forward with long-held plans to expand the hospital's nurses accommodation to cater for a further seventy nurses.

Hospital ambulance service transferred to the Victorian Civil Ambulance Service that year. Describing this development, the jubilee history indulged

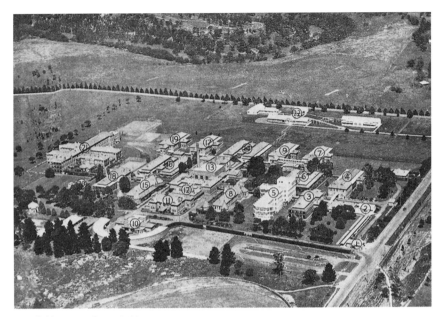

Fairfield Hospital in 1951.

1. Lodge
2. Kiosk and Visitors Guide Room
3. Wards 1 and 2
4. Wards 9 and 10
5. Wards 3, 4 and 5 (F. V. G. Scholes Block)
6. Ward 11
7. Wards 15 and 16
8. Laboratories
9. Wards 17 and 18
10. Garage and Workshop
11. Administrative Block
12. Kitchen and Staff Dining Room
13. Boiler House, Laundries and Stores
14. Wards 19 and 20
15. Wards
16. Wards 12 and 14
17. Wards 21 and 22
18. Wards 6 and 7
19. Wards 23 and 24
20. Lecture Room
21. Nurses' Home
22. Exotic Diseases Unit

in a spot of nostalgia, suggesting that the change was met 'no doubt with the old 'Green Grasshopper' [the affectionate nickname of one of the hospital's first ambulances] nodding sad assent from some ghostly scrap heap'.[5]

In medical terms, 1950/51 recorded a 'record low incidence in the common infectious diseases', but the prevalence of measles, whooping cough and mumps meant that the hospital was keep fairly busy. Poliomyelitis remained a constant problem, with several admissions each week, but numbers remained below epidemic levels. Victoria was indeed fortunate at this time: South Australia was still in the midst of a terrible epidemic which had been raging for over two years, and New South Wales, Queensland and Tasmania had also experienced outbreaks of epidemic proportions. McLorinan, in the 1953 annual report, would have no hesitation in stating that 'Poliomyelitis must be regarded as the most important infectious disease in Australia today'.

An extension to the hospital's resources and services occurred during the year when two 'occupational therapistes', Miss Adam and Miss Middleton, were employed to work with patients in general wards and polio after-care.

The buoyancy and confidence of the Board's post-war annual reports was somewhat deflated in the 1952 annual report. A sombre tone reflected the acute financial difficulties that had beset the hospital: 'It was realised early in the year that any project involving new money would have to be postponed. In addition, the Board closely investigated the financial position, and put into operation measures designed to keep expenditure to the irreducible minimum consistent with safe working.' Clearly a policy based on keeping hospital costs to an 'irreducible minimum' precluded any significant expansion or development of facilities or resources. It is perhaps significant that it was during this period of acute financial stringency that the hospital's annual report first began to incorporate that of the Fairfield Hospital Auxiliary. The stalwart and highly effective work of the Auxiliary was richly deserving of this recognition. One significant development at this time was the reopening, in August 1951, of Wards 23 and 24. These wards, which constituted a 50-bed pavilion, were devoted to patients suffering from pulmonary tuberculosis and were designated as 'the chest unit'.

The opening of the chest unit highlights Fairfield's significant drift away from being a purely a fever hospital, as McLorinan explained in the 1952 annual report:

> The Hospital as at present constituted comprises three divisions—'Fever,' 'General' and 'Chest Unit,' and each division provides interesting medical comparisons in the type of patient treated. The fever division still has the highest admission rate with a rapid turnover of cases. Thus 2071 patients were admitted to this division with an average stay in hospital of 12.2 days. In the general division 1691 patients were admitted with an average stay of 25.7 days. Included in the general division, however, is the after care section for poliomyelitis, in which a number of chronic cases require long term treatment. This unit has provided a valuable service in the care of poliomyelitis in Victoria. Many country cases have been admitted for short periods for the fitting of splints, callipers, etc., and for corrective and physical educational purposes.
>
> The 'chest unit' has admitted 168 cases of pulmonary tuberculosis during the year. Under the care of Dr Renth and with the surgical assistance of Dr Lesley Williams much interesting and valuable work has been performed.
>
> The 'Fever division,' however, remains the most important unit and the individuality of the hospital depends largely on the maintenance of a high standard of medical care, teaching and research in this division.

Clearly McLorinan and the other specialists in infectious diseases on the staff were committed to maintaining the hospital's identity as a 'fever hospital', but

Tuberculosis (TB) Formerly known as consumption or phthisis, TB is caused by the bacillus *Mycobacterium tuberculosis*. Bovine TB (known in England in the Middle Ages as 'scrofula' or the 'King's Evil') is caused by *M. bovis*, which infects cattle and can cause disease in humans. It is transmitted to humans in milk, but this has been controlled in Victoria by eliminating TB in cattle herds and pasteurising milk. In pulmonary tuberculosis a patch of inflammation develops in the lung and an abscess forms. In some cases, there is a rapid spread through both lungs (once described as 'galloping consumption') or the development of miliary tuberculosis. Symptoms include fever, fatigue and night sweats. A chronic cough may develop, with blood-stained sputum. Evidence of TB has been found in Egyptian tombs, dating back to 1000 BCE. The many proposed treatments through the ages have included sleeping in goat stables and drinking asses milk mixed with powdered crab shells. In 1882 Robert Koch in Germany isolated the tubercle bacillus. In 1906 Leon Calmette and Camille Guerin at the Pasteur Institute in Paris started work on a preventative vaccine, and by 1921 had developed the Bacille-Calmette-Guerin (BCG) vaccine.

The first recorded death from TB in Australia was of a crewman of Cook's *Endeavour* in 1770—the first of many thousands. The disease devastated the Aboriginal population as well as the European settlers. The incidence of TB declined steadily in Victoria from the start of the twentieth century, but over the last few decades TB has increasingly become a disease of migrants.

they accepted—given the decreasing demand for fever beds—that the hospital would inevitably have a significant, and in all likelihood increasing, non-infectious diseases component.

The new year brought, as Sandland has noted, 'two momentous happenings' from the hospital's point of view.[6] The first of these was the introduction, for the first time at any fever hospital anywhere in the world, of open visiting. Until this time relatives had only been allowed to visit patients who were well enough to leave the ward. These patients were escorted by staff to a covered Visiting Station—a facility which boasted a wire-netting fence to ensure a separation between patient and visitor and thus contained the infection. The visitor, out in the open and some yards from the patient, was also behind wire netting—with a sort of no-man's land in between. The whole rather unsavoury and demeaning set up was, not surprisingly, known as 'the pens'!

At first, open visiting to the wards was introduced rather pensively (excuse the pun) and experimentally—the hospital was alert for any transmission of infections resulting from this revolutionary initiative. The open visiting proved a great success, and no negative medical repercussions were noted. In the years to come, visiting hours were gradually increased, and it was generally felt that this relaxation played a most positive role in both expediting the physical recovery and promoting the morale of patients and their relatives. The hospital deserves great credit for adopting such an important initiative, which at the time was both novel and risky. Commenting on this development, the jubilee history of the hospital notes:

> The Fairfield hospital is no longer an 'isolation' hospital. Restricted daily visiting is permitted to infectious wards, with visitors suitably gowned as a precautionary measure. The comments of a woman visitor overheard on the path one day seem to sum up the situation: 'When I was a child we darsen't even look in through the fence, we was too frightened, and look at us now![7]

The second milestone of 1952/53, this time in the control of infectious disease, was the introduction of triple antigen. This immunisation, given to babies at two, four, six and eighteen months, provided effective protection from diphtheria, tetanus and whooping cough. Clearly in the years to come this would have a huge impact on hospital admissions and indeed in some ways on the whole complexion of the hospital.

The last graduation ceremony for Fairfield trained nurses took place in 1953. To mark this auspicious and somewhat bittersweet occasion, a Fairfield graduate handed a symbolic torch to a trainee of the Melbourne School of Nursing which, as we have seen, had taken over nursing education.

Poliomyelitis remained the major infectious disease, and the hospital was committed to undertaking as much research into its cause and treatment as its limited resources would allow. Dr Ferris had won a grant from the National Health and Research Council to attend a congress on microbiology in Rome (where he was presenting a paper on leptospirosis) Although the Board of Management was committed to 'rigid economies', it granted finance to Ferris to visit the United Kingdom and the United States to study the latest developments in tissue culture of poliomyelitis virus. Before he left, Ferris supervised important research at the Commonwealth Serum Laboratories, which resulted in poliomyelitis virus from a number of Fairfield patients being cultured in the laboratory. Poliomyelitis remained such a threat to the community that some of the functions organised to mark the first visit of Queen Elizabeth to Australia in 1953 were cancelled due to fears of infection arising from mass gatherings of school children. On a more positive note, a Surgical Unit, a joint project undertaken in association with the Royal Melbourne Hospital and opened in October 1953, marked a significant development in the rapid extension of the hospital's role and functions. The year also saw the publication of the first issue of *Fairfacts*, a monthly magazine for patients and staff devoted to the life of the hospital. This entertaining and informative magazine, largely produced by hospital patients, was to prove a most popular innovation.

The Golden Jubilee of the hospital was celebrated in 1954, and the hospital published a short historical pamphlet entitled *Fairfield Hospital 1904–1954* to mark the occasion. The jubilee was recognised by McLorinan in the 1954 annual report, where he reviewed the changes in fever hospitals since Fairfield was founded. Apart from active service in both world wars, McLorinan had spent his entire professional career treating infectious diseases and administering an infectious disease hospital, having joined the hospital staff in 1919, and his expert comments deserve close attention:

> When the hospital was first founded isolation of the infectious sick with the primary idea of preventing the spread of epidemics was considered as the main function of the hospital. It was soon realised and pointed out by Dr Scholes that this function was of secondary importance and that the main purpose of the hospital was for specialised treatment and the teaching of nurses and medical students.
>
> The period 1920 to 1940 is often spoken of as the golden age of fever hospitals. Large numbers of cases of diphtheria, Scarlet Fever, Measles, Whooping Cough and Meningitis passed through the hospital during this period. Fairfield with its able superintendent, Dr Scholes, achieved a considerable international reputation. We may in retrospect be somewhat critical now of some of the methods used; but the fact remains that an amazing amount of work was carried out with, on the whole, excellent results. It was in fever hospitals that most of then work of isolation and barrier nursing techniques were first propounded and medical asepsis as we know it had its origin in fever hospitals.

After World War II, a marked change in the make-up of fever hospitals occurred, as diphtheria declined dramatically and penicillin greatly reduced the severity of scarlet fever, to such an extent that it could be treated at home. This left fever hospitals with the problem of using empty beds while retaining their skilled staff to deal with epidemics. Fairfield's Board of Management decided that the primary function of the hospital should still be the treatment of acute infective conditions, but that research was also a major consideration, and the hospital laboratory was equipped with the latest laboratory methods of investigation and research into disease prevention and epidemiology. The hospital broadened its admission list to include acute infections known to be transmissible to others, which led to a wide and varied number of acute infections being investigated and treated at Fairfield. More beds were utilised for cases which required diagnosis and investigation as well as treatment. McLorinan wrote:

> In addition as a further service to the community various wards of the hospital have been allotted for other purposes. In 1948, 104 beds were occupied by sub-acute and convalescent medical patients from the Royal Melbourne hospital. Later 50 beds were given over to pulmonary Tuberculosis. A further 60 beds were allocated for the after-care management of Poliomyelitis. A respirator ward in which more and more chronic respirator patients have to be maintained requires a high concentration of nursing staff and physiotherapy personnel. Finally, in October, 1953, a surgical unit of 24 beds was opened for the purpose of reducing the long surgical O.P. waiting list at the Royal Melbourne hospital. We have, therefore, now reached a stage in fever hospital development in which while the primary purpose of the hospital, i.e., the treatment, research and teaching of acute infections is maintained, the hospital is also extending its functions, as a further service to the community.

Unfortunately the jubilee year was marred by the death, on 11 September, of Dr Scholes, Medical Superintendent from 1910 to 1943, who had led the hospital with great success and distinction for almost two-thirds of its fifty years.

A long overdue change took place in the hospital's funding arrangements when the *Infectious Diseases Hospital Act* of 1954 came into operation on 8 February. Under the terms of this Act, municipal councils were no longer required to contribute to the funds of the hospital, the government assuming full financial responsibility through the Hospitals and Charities Fund. The government appointed a new Board of Management of fifteen members in which representation from municipal councils was vastly reduced. It is appropriate now to recognise the great and selfless service that the members of the Board—all of whom were volunteers—had given to the hospital since its inception. The contribution that these men and women had made to the development of the hospital and the health of the community deserves the highest praise. Under the terms of this Act, Queen's Memorial Infectious Diseases hospital was finally 'officially' renamed Fairfield Hospital (having used that name since 1948).

The outstanding contribution that Matron Burbidge had made to nursing in Australia was recognised in 1955 when she was awarded the Order of the British Empire Medal. The year also saw the appointment of Dr E. V. Keogh to the Board. This appointment has been recognised as a 'a very significant milestone' in the development of the hospital. Keogh, a highly decorated World War I veteran, had been a consultant bacteriologist to the

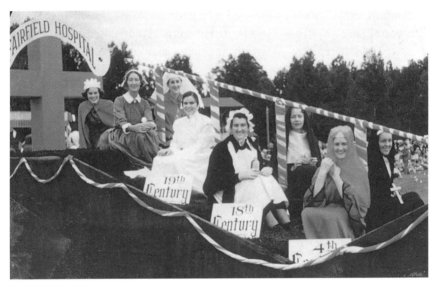

A hospital float in the Australia Day parade of 1955 shows nursing uniforms through the ages.

hospital since 1947 and had won international renown for his scientific research. He had also been Director of Tuberculosis Services in Victoria and Deputy Director of the Commonwealth Serum Laboratories. Keogh was to influence Fairfield Hospital policies and general medical issues in Australia in the years ahead. He energetically encouraged the development of the hospital, and in particular that of the laboratory. His visit to the United States in 1955 expedited the introduction of Salk vaccine into Australia. Keogh's dominance of policies continued until 1961, when he resigned from the Board, but he continued his involvement with the hospital by acting as Consultant Bacteriologist until his death in 1971.

The downward trend in the rate of infectious disease admissions to Fairfield continued. The 1955 annual report stated that poliomyelitis, which had been 'practically an 'endemic' disease' in Melbourne for the previous six years, had been almost absent from Victoria during the winter months—when traditionally the epidemic was at its most severe. Scarlet fever and diphtheria, despite some minor outbreaks, were also markedly lower than would have been expected. A severe epidemic of whooping cough resulted in the admission of 293 patients—most of whom were severely affected—with a relatively low death rate of 1.35 per cent. In earlier years mortality rates of over 20 per cent had been the norm. This remarkable improvement was due to the use of broad spectrum antibiotics, which proved most effective in diminishing the severity of pulmonary complications that had so often led to death in the past.

Two of the most common reasons for admission—gastro-intestinal infections and infective hepatitis—were from outside the 'traditional' diseases admitted to the hospital. There were 214 admissions for gastro-intestinal infections—by far the largest number in the history of the hospital—primarily of patients suffering from Sonne dysentery, and 193 admissions for infective hepatitis, again by far the highest recorded number for this disease. The year was also notable in that a virus laboratory was established in a 'small room in the main laboratory'.

Sir Albert Coates was elected chair of the Board of Management in 1956. He continued as chair for seventeen years, making an outstanding contribution to the development of the hospital. Sir Albert's perception of the hospital's role was very much in line with the thinking of Dr McLorinan. In his first year as chair, and on numerous other occasions, he stated that its function was not only to treat infectious patients and to maintain facilities for epidemic periods, but also to perform epidemiological studies and research. The importance of having a progressive Board, prepared to support the expert opinions and planning objectives of senior medical staff, can hardly be overstated.

Hepatitis may be caused by any of a number of related viruses. The symptoms result from damage caused to cells of the liver by the virus, and the consequent decrease in liver function. Infection usually results in low-grade fever, malaise, nausea, abdominal pain and jaundice. Many cases of hepatitis are so mild that a person may be unaware of infection. Fulminant hepatitis is a life-threatening infection that results in severe liver failure, impaired kidney function, difficulty in the clotting of blood, and marked changes in neurological function. The first description of hepatitis has been attributed to the Hippocratic School in the second century BCE. In the 1960s the virus causing hepatitis B was isolated, and a successful vaccine was developed in the 1970s. There is also now an effective vaccine for preventing hepatitis A.

Sir Albert Coates (1895–1977) was born in Ballarat on 28 January 1895. He began working at the age of eleven and educated himself by attending night classes. He served at Gallipoli and France during World War I and, when repatriated, worked at night and studied medicine at the University of Melbourne during the day—winning first-class honours despite his difficult circumstances. He worked in various hospitals and lectured in anatomy at the University of Melbourne (1925–40), specialising in neurosurgery.

During World War II Coates rejoined the army and went to Malaya with the AIF in 1941. He was captured by the Japanese at Sumatra in 1942 and spent the rest of the war in prisoner-of-war camps in Sumatra, Burma and Thailand. His name is forever linked with that of Edward 'Weary' Dunlop for the magnificent medical work they performed under the most primitive and barbaric of conditions.

Coates retired in 1971 but remained active in medical and community organisations. (See Coates and Rosenthal, *The Albert Coates Story*).

The hospital was honoured at this time to be selected to test the safety of the Salk vaccine produced in Australia, and shortly after these successful tests the Commonwealth Serum Laboratories started producing Salk vaccine to combat poliomyelitis infections. This vaccine, prepared by US physician Jonas E. Salk, was one of the most important medical advances of the century and was, of course, of particular importance to those working in infectious diseases hospitals. The significance of vaccine for the community at large and for the hospital is shown by the fact that the artificial ventilation requirements of polio patients had caused Fairfield to establish one of the world's largest tank respirator (iron lung) wards. It is also worth noting that hepatitis became a notifiable disease during the year.

In the 1957 annual report, McLorinan was able to record an 'extraordinary reduction in the incidence of poliomyelitis'. He cautioned, however, that it was still 'too early to be sanguine that this is solely due to the intensive Salk campaign which has been carried out successfully in Victoria'. Despite his professional caution he was nonetheless optimistic, noting that 'it would appear likely, as happened with diphtheria, that if a sufficient proportion of children of school age are immunised, the disease will cease to be a threat to adults'. McLorinan also drew attention to the fact that diphtheria and scarlet fever, which had led in the past to the greatest proportion of admissions, were now relatively insignificant. In explaining this dramatic change he noted that 'Bacterial infections are not now the dominant cause for Admissions to hospitals such as Fairfield. Antibiotics and immunisation procedures have been the main cause of this change.' This welcome alleviation in many of the diseases that had caused so much suffering and death over the centuries did not mean that the hospital was becoming redundant, as McLorinan pointed out:

> On the other hand, virus diseases as a cause of hospital admissions show a proportional increase. The main increases have occurred in infective hepatitis and virus infections of the central nervous system. But if we include some of the respiratory infections as of virus origin the proportional increase becomes more marked.

As we shall see, McLorinan's analysis of the growing importance of virus diseases was to be most amply and tragically proven in the following decades.

A new strain of influenza descended on Australia in late June 1957. Dubbed 'Asian flu', this virus infected an estimated 500 000 Victorians, with 672 victims being admitted to Fairfield, 38 of whom lost their lives. This epidemic was the worst to hit Melbourne since the infamous Spanish flu pandemic in 1918–19. It was a difficult time for the hospital for, as Sandland has noted, 'the most worrying times are those when the virus undergoes major changes or 'shifts' in antigenicity, such as the appearance of the 'Asian' strain in 1957'.[8] This epidemic was followed soon after by epidemics of viral meningitis and infectious hepatitis.

On 14 November 1957 the Minister for Health re-opened Ward 12, which had been renovated to accommodate 'old' poliomyelitis patients who required prolonged artificial respiration. Many of these long-term patients came to see Fairfield as their second home and became recognised as notable characters around the hospital. The heroic efforts they made to live as normal a life as possible provided inspiration to other patients and hospital staff. During the year the Victorian Associated Brewers presented a Volkswagen bus to the hospital for the use of poliomyelitis patients. The bus, which was fitted out with respirator bellows and other important adaptations, was used to take them on recreational outings and other visits, significantly improving the quality of life of many who had previously been unable to leave the hospital. In a similar vein the donation of television sets to the children's wards by the *Herald* newspaper was extremely popular, although whether television improved the quality of life on the children's wards is perhaps debatable.

Matron Burbidge reported in 1958 that the shortage of trained nursing staff and the (long overdue) adoption of a 40-hour week and straight 8-hour

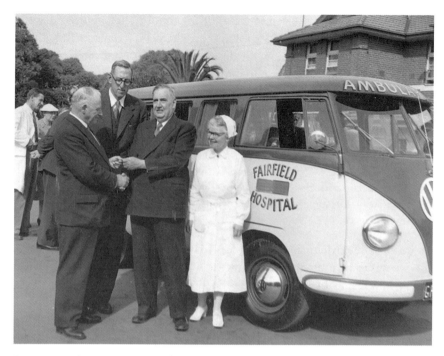

Mr Fogarty of Victorian Associated Brewers presents the keys of a new bus to Sir Albert Coates, Chairman of the Board of Management (left), watched by Mr Coleman and Matron Burbidge, May 1957.

shifts for nurses had been tackled by increasing the number of nursing aides employed and by employing untrained ward helpers. This was not, of course, an ideal resolution of the hospital's staffing difficulties, and Matron Burbidge drew attention to the added burden on trained staff due to the increased numbers of untrained staff and the constantly changing rotations of student nurses.

The sterling work that Fairfield had undertaken during the influenza epidemic provided Dr McLorinan with the opportunity to answer those in the medical fraternity and political spheres who questioned the necessity—and indeed the wisdom—of having a specialised infectious diseases hospital. McLorinan in the 1958 annual report noted that:

> The wisdom of the policy of retaining Fairfield hospital as a special hospital primarily for the treatment of infectious diseases has been apparent in recent years. Despite optimistic forecasts from some quarters, the demand continues for beds for the investigation and treatment of patients suffering from infectious diseases from both the city and country. In the past three years there have been major epidemics of infectious hepatitis, virus meningitis (E.C.H.O. and Cox-

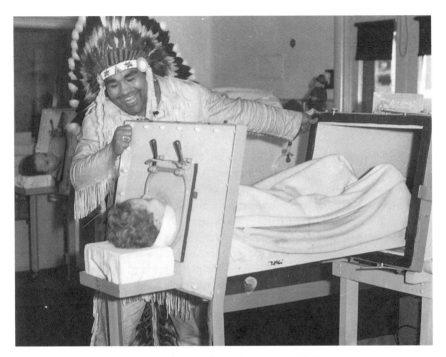

Big Chief LittleWolf visits a child in an old-style respirator, 1958.

sackie), Asian Influenza, and minor outbreaks of whooping cough, measles and other common diseases. There is now a minor outbreak of poliomyelitis, which may develop into a major outbreak. Fairfield accommodated a vast majority of patients who were severely affected in these epidemics. In addition there is a continuous demand for beds for acute infections such as meningitis both bacterial and viral, encephalitis, tetanus, obstructive laryngitis and pneumonia. At one time recently, patients suffering from twelve different varieties of meningitis were being treated. These acute infections are referred to Fairfield for diagnosis and treatment, not only by private practitioners, but also by the large teaching hospitals, who rely on the consultative capacity of the hospital which is derived from the experience of the permanent medical staff using special facilities in the wards and laboratories. Fairfield plays a major role in conjunction with the Health Department in the control of communicable diseases in Victoria. The Epidemiological Unit is the intelligence service for such control.

It must have been galling for McLorinan and the other specialist and deeply committed staff of the hospital that there was a perennial need to plead the hospital's case, or perhaps more accurately 'fight the hospital's corner'. The need to defend the hospital's role and indeed its very existence was to remain a constant underlying pressure over the succeeding years.

The Board meanwhile, still operating under the 'strictest economy', was fighting an uphill battle to maintain the standard of the hospital's buildings and facilities. It was hoping that somehow a plan could be put in place which would solve the hospital's resource problems. This was discussed in the 1958 annual report:

> The reconstruction of Ward 12 was the first major building work undertaken for many years, and the Board is at present engaged in formulating a policy for presentation to the hospitals and Charities Commission to bring the hospital generally up to modern standards. In the meantime, it is hoped that other wards, which fall short of requirements, can be similarly improved. Many of our wards, which were built in the main for children suffering from diphtheria and scarlet fever, are now needed for treatment of other diseases and for rehabilitation purposes, lack the essential requirements for these activities. Unfortunately, limited finance was available and necessary improvements have had to be deferred, but it is hoped that a plan will be adopted which will ensure that in the immediate future years some of the more urgent work will be undertaken.

The financial problems referred to by the Board, and the tendency in some quarters to question the continued need for a specialised infectious diseases hospital, were not unrelated. Governments of whatever political complexion are unwilling to invest in an institution which might be past its use-by date.

In the 1959 annual report the Board continued to challenge the argument that there was no longer any need for specialised infectious diseases hospitals such as Fairfield. Those who questioned the continuation of the hospital argued that all infectious diseases hospitals had been rendered redundant by medical advances rather than advancing any individual critique of the performance of Fairfield. As the Board said, 'Unfortunately, an impression has been gained in many quarters that infectious diseases are not as prevalent these days, and that, therefore, the function of the hospital should be changed'. In answer, the Board simply echoed—more or less word for word—McLorinan's powerfully argued defence which had appeared in the previous year's annual report. The Board was, however, in a position to state that both the Department of Health and the Hospitals and Charities Commission had recognised the importance of Fairfield's specialised role, and that 'a firm agreement' had been reached that 'any development of the hospital should be in line with its primary specialist function, i.e., the diagnosis and treatment of infectious diseases'. In order to expedite the future development of the hospital's resources and services, the Board established a special Medical Advisory Committee under Sir Albert Coates—who was also chair of the Board of

Management. All of the Board's hopes and plans were, of course, as nothing unless government funding was forthcoming.

Commenting upon the huge variety of infectious diseases treated at Fairfield during 1958/59, McLorinan was forced to conclude that Fairfield's 'table of admissions' illustrated the 'formidable number of communicable virus diseases prevalent in the community'. Indeed with 5000 admissions, Fairfield had experienced its busiest year for some time. A localised polio-myelitis outbreak in a northern suburb in July 1958, and more particularly a recurrence of Asian influenza (which in this instance primarily affected the older age group), were factors in creating the unusually high demands on the hospital. Due to lack of funding, some of the old fever wards had fallen into a state of disrepair, so the hospital found it impossible to open the reserve fever wards and was forced to access beds from the Royal Melbourne Hospital convalescent section and the After-care and Rehabilitation Units. Clearly this was not an ideal situation.

One positive development in 1959 was the transfer of the tuberculosis laboratory—which had been sited at the hospital since 1947—from the control of the University of Melbourne to Fairfield Hospital. This trend to concentration of public health functions at Fairfield was to be extended in later years. The centralising of infectious disease research reflected the wide-spread recognition that Fairfield had unsurpassed experience and expertise in the field of infectious diseases.

The final year of the decade saw the last serious outbreak of polio-myelitis in Victoria. The near eradication of this dreadful and terrifying disease was a triumph for the effectiveness of Salk's polio vaccine. The hospital was not, of course, finished with poliomyelitis as it continued to be involved with the care of polio victims until the day it closed.

It is fitting to end the decade with a highlight, and one can think of few more uplifting things for the staff of a hospital than the thanks of parents whose child has been restored to health. For the first time in the hospital's history, the 1959 annual report saw fit to publish one of the many appreci-ative letters that the hospital received each year. From the father of a 6-year-old boy, it is an example of the impact that Fairfield had on so many lives over the years:

> Dear Sir,
>
> Now that we are settling back into a more normal routine following our little boy's discharge from your hospital, I would like to take just a few moments in writing and expressing our sincere thanks to you and your staff. I remember clearly the form which I was required to sign when we picked John up just two weeks ago. One question there simply asked—'Are you satisfied with the treat-

ment he has received?' To merely answer in the affirmative seemed to be totally inadequate, but I feel that I now have an opportunity on behalf of myself and my wife to elaborate on that answer.

From the very first moment that we entered Fairfield for the first time we were met everywhere with kindness, consideration and efficiency. From the main entrance where the lodge-keepers were very courteous and helpful at all times, right through the hospital and out again we were met with the same kindness and consideration.

We wish to extend to all the medical officers, the wonderful team of Sisters and nurses, our very sincere thanks for all that they have done and are doing. We know that you all insist that 'it is your job', and to an extent that is so, but the way all your staff carry out that job carries it much further than just an occupation. Although we have been through a very worrying and anxious time, we are grateful to God for the experience of coming to meet and know so many at 'Fairfield' and its staff, and others like it and pray that His rich blessings be upon you all.

It is important as we examine the history of the hospital that we pause every so often to reflect upon the real life dramas, joys and tragedies which make up the day-to-day life of a major infectious diseases hospital. Generations of Melbourne folk have viewed the hospital with great respect and affection, tinged with fear, for infectious diseases are extremely frightening to

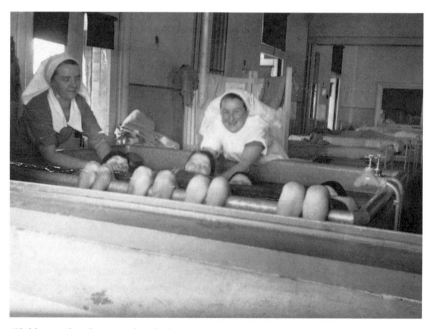

Children with polio in a saline bath

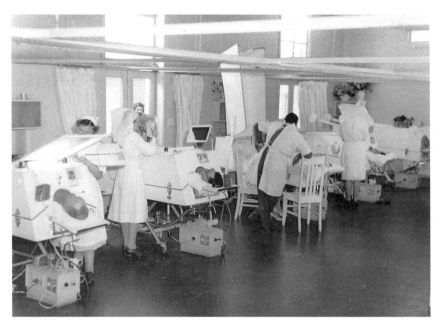

Polio patients in Ward 12, 1960.

the general public. There can be few, if any, Victorian families who have not at some time had cause to be grateful for the expert care and humanity which the hospital provided.

The hospital entered the 1960s—a tumultous and troubled decade—basking in the praise of Dr Hattie Alexander, an eminent paediatrician and world renowned authority on infectious diseases. Alexander, who visited Australia with the assistance of a Felton Bequest, spent some time at Fairfield and was lavish in her praise. The Board published two letters from Alexander in the 1960 annual report:

> I want you to know how impressed I am with the high calibre of the staff at Fairfield and the work they are doing. It seems to me that you are one of the rare good institutions still specialising in infectious diseases. While there has been a valid reason for the present trend of absorbing patients with infectious diseases in general hospitals some important assets have been lost. Most infectious disease hospitals in the past were staffed with doctors who are not top flight. As a result patients often failed to receive the best care and new advances in our knowledge in this field did not evolve. At Fairfield hospital your clinicians are top flight people and those who are engaged in laboratory investigations are making significant contributions. I know of no other hospital so well equipped for defining viral etiologic agents. I hope you will use your influence to keep

Fairfield intact as an institute for study of infectious diseases. I shall look forward to receiving publications from Fairfield.

Dr McLorinan described Alexander's visit to the hospital as the 'most important event of the hospital year 1959/60'. He received a personal letter from her in which she said:

> The time I spent at Fairfield hospital let me know that you are doing a superb job there both in clinical and investigational medicine. I think you are one of the few places in the world in which there are still opportunities to increase our understanding of infectious diseases by study of the patients themselves as well as laboratory aspects.

Given the difficult struggle that McLorinan and his staff had had in realising his vision of Fairfield as a centre of excellence in treatment of and research into infectious diseases, the high praise heaped on the hospital and its staff by Alexander was not only extremely gratifying but was also a resounding vindication of the hospital's existence.

From the early 1960s the annual admission rate began to increase again. Critical factors in this resurgence of infectious disease were the increasing child population—which had almost doubled since 1947—the occurrence of new epidemic problems, and improved transport facilities enabling the admission of more patients from country districts. While this trend was clearly problematic for the hospital it did, to some extent, help to ensure its continuation.

Two major changes took place in 1960. G. N. Burbidge, who had been Matron since 1939, retired. A description of her in the seventy-fifth anniversary edition of the annual report noted that she was 'a dainty person, a strict disciplinarian and, along with Dr Scholes was instrumental in laying the foundations for today's infectious disease nursing procedures'. Her replacement was Vivien Bullwinkel, whose dramatic and heroic military record and reputation as a nurse were well known throughout Australia. The hospital counted itself extremely fortunate to have obtained the services of such an outstanding new Matron.

The second major change was the retirement of Henry McLorinan, who had been appointed Medical Superintendent in 1948. Earlier in 1960 McLorinan had been created a CBE, and had been elected president of the Australian Paediatric Association (now known as the Australian College of Paediatrics). McLorinan had made a huge contribution to the hospital over many years—a good deal of the credit for the dramatic expansion of the hospital's research role, for example, belonged to him. Dr John Allan Forbes was appointed to replace McLorinan. Forbes—who interrupted his medical studies to serve with the 2nd AIF in World War II and was one of the famed

'Rats of Tobruk'—had been attached to the hospital since 1949 and Deputy Superintendent since 1954. He has been described as a 'very determined' man 'of great personal charm' who 'believed that principles overrode details'.

The year also saw Sir Macfarlane Burnet, Fairfield's Honorary Consultant Epidemiologist, sharing the Nobel Prize for Medicine and Physiology with Sir Peter Medawar, for research on acquired immunological tolerance to tissue transplants. Burnet had made a great contribution to research into infectious diseases, having previously discovered how to identify bacteria by the viruses (bacteriophages) that attack them, and had developed a technique of culturing viruses in living chick embryos.

The most significant factor in the pattern of admissions for 1960/61 was the continued growth in admissions of patients suffering from communicable diseases. From a low point in 1954 when only 2077 fever patients were admitted, the number had grown steadily to a near record 4913. This figure was inflated by two major epidemics of bronchiolitis in infants. These epidemics—caused by the then recently recognised respiratory syncytial virus—led to an extremely high rate of admissions and, given the continuing shortage of trained nursing staff, put the hospital under considerable pressure.

The pattern of increasing admissions of infectious disease patients continued into 1961/62. In the 1962 annual report, Forbes described the increase and reflected upon its causes:

> The increase in the demand for beds for communicable diseases at this hospital over the last ten years has been maintained during the year 1st July, 1961 to 30th June 1962, with the admission of 5,702 fever patients. This number is equivalent to the largest previous years in 1932 and 1936 when the admissions were dominated by diphtheria and scarlet fever. During the year, diverse epidemics including measles, infective hepatitis, enterovirus, meningitis, whooping cough, varicella, mumps, tonsillitis and pharyngitis, gastro-enteritis and respiratory virus infections, have given rise to the bulk of these patients.
>
> The current average stay of patients in hospital of 13 days contrasts with that of 15 or more years ago when it was commonly longer than 30 days; consequently the requisite number of hospital beds for communicable diseases has been correspondingly reduced. It has been assessed by this hospital in conjunction with the Commission of Public Health of Victoria that a specialised hospital for Communicable Diseases in Melbourne (a well-immunised population of about 1,900,000) requires 300 active beds with an available reserve of 150 beds.
>
> The severe and complicated cases of various epidemic diseases in general are admitted to Fairfield hospital so that admissions reflect to a large extent the epidemic state of Melbourne and to some extent, Victoria. The concentration of these cases makes possible the provision of specialised facilities for their investigation and management and the integration of clinical and laboratory aspects which is so desirable in elucidating infective problems. This is illustrated

by the fact that the results of investigation of specimens derived outside the hospital are disappointing compared to those within the hospital and argues against the principle of decentralisation of patients and the establishment of central laboratories remote from patients and clinicians. Also, the capacity to study a full range of infective disease is important for clinical comparison and the assessment of casual relationship between the various agents and diseases in question.

The first of two other major events for the year was the laying of the foundation stone for the new and much-needed Albert Coates Block for Medical Services. Construction of the building, which was to house a pharmacy, radiology unit, central sterile supply facility, lecture rooms and an operating theatre, was commenced on 18 June 1962. The building was named in honour of Sir Albert Coates, in recognition of his long years of dedicated service to the hospital. It was officially opened by the Minister for Health, R. W. Mack, on 21 March 1963. The building, which was designed by the architect Hugh Peck and Partners, received a great deal of praise—particularly for the unique way in which it was designed in order to centralise so many different hospital functions.

The other major event was that Fairfield became affiliated with the recently opened Monash University. Monash, like the University of Melbourne which had been associated with Fairfield since 1905, wanted its medical students to receive specialised instruction in infectious diseases at Fairfield. As it was fifth-year medical students who undertook a residence at Fairfield, the first students did not come to the hospital until 1965.

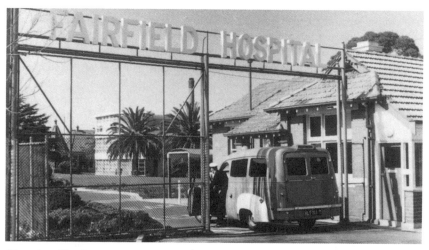

The prison-like front gate in 1960.

Commenting in the 1962 annual report on this development and on the importance of the hospital's educational role, Forbes noted that:

Teaching is a natural adjunct to the primary function of the hospital not only in the demonstration of individual patients but also of their place in the patterns of epidemic disease in the community and their relation to the problems of preventive medicine and public health. In demonstrating communicable diseases that are acute, rapidly changing and transient, it is desirable to provide continuity of observation. The response to antibiotic treatment of various bacterial diseases, too, is so rapid that unless students are present when the patient is admitted much of the lesson, particularly in the management of simple, lethal complications such as vomiting in the comatose patient, is lost. To obviate this, Monash students will reside in the hospital for periods of two or three weeks so that the course of the various communicable diseases can be observed and procedures of investigation and management fully appreciated and practiced.

Infectious disease admissions reached 5928 in 1962/63. This increase was attributed to the changing pattern of epidemic diseases, increases in the population and advances in techniques of investigation and treatment. Epidemics of diphtheria and measles also contributed. This was to be the last major diphtheria outbreak in Victoria, with 141 cases admitted to the hospital. There were no fatalities from the diphtheria epidemic and this once killer disease would never again cause a patient's death at the hospital. The measles epidemic, which commenced in April 1963 and peaked in August, led to 758 admissions. It was thought to have been 'the largest epidemic of measles yet experienced in Melbourne', the upward trend being seen as related to the increasing number of children in the community.

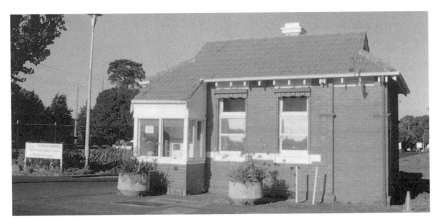

And the same gate in 1990.

Sir Macfarlane Burnet was born in Traralgon on 3 September 1899. While working as resident pathologist at Melbourne hospital he became interested in bacterial viruses, and completed a PhD at London University and research at the Lister Institute in 1927.

On returning to Australia he was appointed assistant director of the Walter and Eliza Hall Institute. In 1931 with Jean Macnamara he discovered that there were at least two strains of the poliomyelitis virus. He discovered the organism which caused Q fever in 1935—named *Coxiella burnetti* in recognition of his work. During World War II he experimented on influenza vaccine with soldiers.

Appointed Director of the Walter and Eliza Hall Institute and Professor of Experimental Medicine at the University of Melbourne in 1994, he established the Clinical Research Unit in 1946, to serve as a bridge between the Institute and the clinical work at the Melbourne hospital. He continued to study virology until 1957 when he began to focus on immunology. In a paper entitled 'The Production of Antibodies' published in 1949 Burnet had proposed a theory of acquired immunological tolerance (in other words, that disease was not inevitable as inoculation against viruses could prevent the attack of antibodies). Peter Medawar, an English immunologist, proved Burnet's hypothesis in 1951.

Burnet made important contributions to knowledge about virus diseases such as Murray Valley fever (which the Murray Valley tourism lobby requested be renamed Australian fever). Burnet injected himself with the myxoma virus to show that an outbreak in the Mildura area was not linked to the spread of myxomatosis by mosquitoes. Wide international acclaim included the Royal Society's Royal and Copley medals, the Mueller medal and the Order of the Rising Sun. He also received honorary doctorates from Oxford and Cambridge universities. A prolific writer, Burnet's books include *Viruses and Man* (1955), *Integrity and the Body* (1962), *Self and Not-Self* (1969), *Dominant Mammal* (1970) and *Natural History of Infectious Diseases* (1972). Burnet turned down many prestigious invitations, preferring to live and work in Australia. (See Sexton, *Burnet,* and *Medical Journal of Australia* 143 (12/13) 1985.)

The intense pressure placed on the hospital by the extremely high level of admissions was compounded by the closure of the Victorian School of Nursing during the year. In an attempt to alleviate the shortage of nursing staff, Fairfield established its own Nursing Aide Training School—an initiative which was so successful that by June 1963 the new training school started to accept students from other hospitals. The hospital received a huge feather in its cap during the year when it was designated as a World Health Organisation Influenza Centre. As a result of this prestigious affiliation the Virus Laboratory at Fairfield developed a close collaboration with the Virus Unit of the World Health Organisation. In 1964 the World Health Organisation again honoured Fairfield when it designated the hospital's laboratory as the Oceanic Regions Reference Centre for Enteroviruses and Respiratory Viruses.

In 1964/65 the hospital admitted 6880 patients, of whom no less than 6763 were defined as acute fever patients. Clearly the days when the hospital had been forced to accept 'overflow' patients from other hospitals in order to keep its beds filled were long gone. One of the most challenging—and scientifically interesting—diseases treated during the year was a major epidemic of Coxsackie Virus Type B5. This previously relatively rare virus reached epidemic proportions in Melbourne during the summer, with 287 victims admitted. The virus also caused an increase in pericarditis and myocarditis and this also led to a number of admissions.

The Board of Management, which had been examining the medical staffing of the hospital for some time, appointed four additional regular visiting medical specialists in 1966—a general physician, a paediatrician, a neurologist and a haematologist. Although only part-time, these specialist appointments constituted a significant addition to the hospital's resources. The hospital's expanding role as a specialist training centre again increased in February 1966 when trainee nurses from Repatriation General Hospital started to attend Fairfield for paediatric nursing experience. The year also saw the physiotherapy school, which had been housed at the hospital for many years, transfer to new quarters in central Melbourne (Swanston Street).

In his contribution to the annual report in 1966, Forbes quoted a statement by Rene Dubos in his recent book, *Man Adapting* :

> Most clinicians, public health officers, epidemiologists and microbiologists felt justified ... in proclaiming during the 1950s that the conquest of infectious diseases had finally been achieved. The deans of medical schools and their faculties had so little doubt on the subject that they made it a practice (and still continue!) to appoint to the chairs of medical microbiology biochemists or geneticists essentially unconcerned with the mechanisms of infectious processes.

Surprisingly enough this euphoria has not yet been dampened by the fact that the morbidity rates of infection have not decreased significantly, and in some cases have actually increased.

Forbes went on to analyse trends at Fairfield.

Considerable confusion in attitudes to the importance of infectious diseases has been created by assuming that the reduction in mortality indicates a reduction in morbidity. Indeed, the reduction in mortality is maintained to a large extent by improved facilities for treatment rather than a change in the nature of a disease. The list of diseases admitted to the hospital during the 1930s is akin to the present list but the distribution has changed in some respects. Gastro-enteritis and hepatitis have superseded diphtheria and scarlet fever as the dominant public health diseases and some agents, formerly anonymous, have been identified so

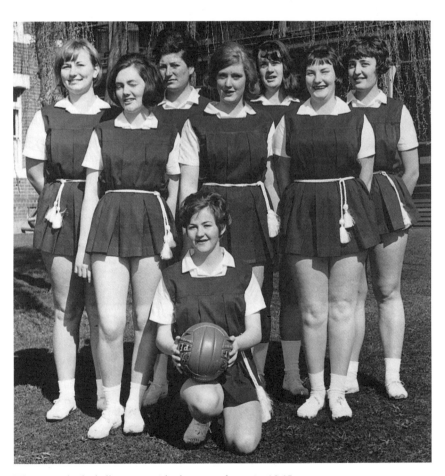

The nurses basketball team outside the nurses home in 1965.

that a new nomenclature has appeared to change the time-honoured diseases which have always contributed large numbers of severe and complicated cases during the recurring epidemic periods.

Following a visit to the hospital in March 1966, the distinguished epidemiologist, Professor Thomas Anderson, from the Department of Epidemiology and Preventive Medicine at the University of Glasgow in Scotland, wrote an extremely complimentary (and at times prophetic) letter of commendation and analysis to the hospital. Anderson's letter was so positive about the hospital and its long-term role and importance that the Board of Management cast modesty to the winds and printed it in its entirety in the 1966 annual report. The letter read in part:

> You will appreciate that the name of Fairfield was already well known to me before I came to Australia. I have always regarded it as one of the important world centres for the study of communicable disease and I knew that in coming to it I would myself be the recipient of much stimulus and encouragement. This indeed proved to be the case, and I can assure you that in the various meetings and discussions a great deal of ground was covered and valuable information interchanged. If any assurance from me were necessary then you can take it that Fairfield is in good heart.
>
> It has been only too easy in recent years, as one after another of the great pestilences of the past has been brought under control, to imagine that all the best work has now been done and that the need for such hospitals is past. You can understand that I have given much thought to this over the years, and I have tried to be as objective in my approach as possible. The fact is that hospitals like Fairfield have an important role even in modern times. In the foreseeable future man is unlikely to reach a time when microbiological agents fail to make their impact on him. What will happen is that the diseases will change. Each new period will produce environmental alterations which will in turn alter the bacteria and viruses with which man must come to terms. It may be that the enormous numbers of cases and deaths which made the plagues of the past so fearsome will not be repeated; but infection and man's response to it still require intensive study. Those who work at Fairfield are making significant contributions in this field.

Professor Anderson's comments were not, however, wholly complimentary: he did draw attention to the fact that the hospital's laboratory, housed as it was in re-designed wards, badly needed to be replaced by a specially designed laboratory facility.

After years of frustration a new ward block for the care of young children and babies was built in 1967. It speaks volumes for the poor resourcing of the hospital that this was the first new ward accommodation for eighteen years. The new two-storey block provided 63 isolation beds with good visibility for observation and non-circulating air-conditioning (with corridor pressures positive relative to that in the cubicles), which greatly lessened the risk of cross-infection. The new block also contained a tracheotomy theatre with three steam rooms, four large solaria and play spaces on the northern verandahs of each floor. Named the Henry McLorinan Block, it was officially opened on 29 June 1967 by the Minister for Health, V. O. Dickie.

Fairfield's Medical Superintendent, Dr J. A. Forbes, joined one of the civilian medical teams in Vietnam for a period of ten weeks under the auspices of the Department of External Affairs in February 1967. This visit helped the hospital to extend its interests, particularly in the field of tropical diseases, and paved the way for Fairfield to become a reference centre for tropical diseases with facilities for their treatment. In April, Fairfield was honoured to host combined meeting of the Preventive Medicine Society and the Scientific Branch of the Australian Medical Association. The introduction of the national Sabin oral poliomyelitis vaccine program on 1 May was welcomed by the hospital community. The hospital still cared for a number of the victims of earlier poliomyelitis outbreaks, and staff tirelessly promoted and supported any preventive measures taken to reduce the risk of further outbreaks of this devastating disease.

Early in 1968 the hospital significantly extended the times during which patients could be visited. The new arrangements proved most popular with visitors and patients. Staff felt that children in particular derived great benefit from the increased contact with family and friends, helping to reduce the inevitable problems associated with separation from the family whist hospitalised. This extension of visiting hours was part of a general liberalisation of hospital rules and regulations that was to gain pace in the following years.

The Deputy Medical Superintendent, Dr N. Bennett, joined a medical team in Vietnam for eleven weeks in August 1967. As a result of Bennett's overseas service, the Department of External Affairs (under whose auspices Bennett's visit was made) entered into discussions with Fairfield about the hospital undertaking a diseases survey of Australian medical teams in Vietnam. Largely due to the enthusiasm and efforts of Dr Forbes and the assistance of local heraldry experts, in 1969 the hospital acquired its own coat of arms. The first of the new badges incorporating the coat of arms were presented to nursing staff soon after it was granted. On a less pleasant note the year also saw the Board being forced to object to plans for the proposed siting of the controversial new Eastern Freeway. The original plans, which the Board found objectionable, significantly encroached on hospital land.

As Fairfield moved towards the end of the 1960s Forbes warned that 'The alleged conquest of infectious diseases is somewhat illusory in that the reduction in mortalities does not reflect the persistent high morbidity figures from infection nor the necessity to continue specialised work to retain control of the existing situation'. This warning was indeed timely. Sandland drew attention to the profound impact that these developments had on Fairfield:

> Mention should be made of diseases associated with changing habits and standards in our community. In 1969 some Melbourne drug users shared syringes with Sydney friends and became jaundiced and ill. That year it became possible to identify in patients the marker of Hepatitis B, the agent of long incubation disease principally seen prior to that time as a hazard of mass inoculation and particularly from blood transfusions. But now the drug culture had arrived, and to a certain extent the character of the whole hospital was altered, with the advent of a large number of disturbed young devotees with Hepatitis B of varying severity, and also the setting up of a Dialysis Unit at the hospital to treat Hepatitis B carriers who had chronic renal failure . . . While the incidence of Hepatitis B is largely bound up with drug takers, though certain migrant groups have high carrier rates, its incidence is also as a result of the Sexual Revolution, as, of course is the recent vast recrudescence in Venereal Disease. Fairfield hospital as an institution is only on the fringe of the action here . . .[9]

Fairfield may still have been 'on the fringe of the action' as the decade drew to a close, but in the last quarter-century of the hospital's history we will see that it was to move into centre stage as new developments in infectious diseases presented tremendous—and previously unimagined—challenges.

Progress and Challenge
1970–1985

> We think that the policy of centralising infectious diseases treatment at Fairfield Hospital is a sound one, and that with diseases of this nature, particularly those that occur only rarely or periodically, a dispersal of expertise is to be avoided.
>
> *Report . . . into Hospital and Health Services in Victoria, 1976.*[1]

SIGNIFICANT CHANGES IN the senior staff at Fairfield took place in 1970, with Dr Allan Ferris (Microbiologist) resigning to accept a senior appointment at Monash University and Dr Ian Gust joining the staff as a Medical Virologist—over the next decade Gust was to make the Virology Department at Fairfield one of the best of its kind in the world and establish himself as a world authority in his field of expertise. On 22 June, former Medical Superintendent Dr Henry McLorinan died. His name had been for many years been synonymous with Fairfield Hospital, and his association with the hospital spanned half a century. Although he had retired from the Superintendent's position on 31 December 1960, he remained a consultant to the hospital until the time of his death. As well as his commitments to Fairfield, McLorinan was also a longstanding member of the Commission of Public Health, Victoria. During his long and distinguished career, McLorinan won a reputation both within Australia and on the international stage as an eminent authority on infectious diseases.

The establishment of the Hospital and Allied Services Advisory Council, an organisation designed to advise on co-ordination of hospitals and services, was a positive start to the new decade, as was the introduction of the measles immunisation campaign. This campaign used vaccine supplied by the Commonwealth Serum Laboratories and was so successful that by 1972 all Australian states were participating. Another campaign instituted at this time was directed towards resolving the perennial problem of shortage of nursing staff. As part of this campaign the hospital, assisted by M. F. Lucy, a member of the Board, produced a brochure designed to be 'distributed widely as a means of augmenting our staff'.

144

Remodelling of Ward 14 commenced in May 1970, and was completed the following year. The new ward was designed to be a specialised facility for patients with acute respiratory infections, and for those requiring respirators. The ward was also designed to provide facilities for treatment of haemo-dialysis patients—'for whom, under certain conditions, admission has been requested from time to time'.

The hospital, like many areas of Melbourne, was affected by freeway development and lodged a complaint against the proposed route of the Eastern Freeway. The 1970 Annual Report recorded success:

> The Formal Objection to the proposed siting of the new Eastern Freeway, which was submitted by the Board because of the serious effects this would have on the functioning of the hospital, was heard in October, 1969. It is pleasing to report that the Objection was allowed and that the Freeway will be sited south of the hospital boundary away from ward buildings. The Board records its appreciation of the special interest and valuable services of Mr. Lucy and Mr. Donaldson in relation to this problem.

Recently returned from a tour of duty in Vietnam, the Medical Super-intendent, Dr John Forbes, presented in the 1970 annual report an incisive and at times prophetic analysis of the role and importance of a specialised infectious diseases hospital:

> In addition to the admission of over 6,000 acute patients requiring hospital management, the provision of special clinics for specific problems such as rubella and hepatitis, investigation of field outbreaks, the testing of numerous specimens from patients in other hospitals and at home, including the screening of sera for specialised service in a community in which the 'conquest' of infectious diseases is claimed. Such 'conquests' in both preventive and curative fields are largely illusory and are certainly not self-perpetuating. The need for specialised facilities to enable precision in diagnosis, specialised patient care and the maintenance of a specific surveillance service is increased by suppression of some epidemic diseases which become a covert threat.

Several unexpected outbreaks during the year had been a reminder that infectious diseases could emerge at any time. The first bacteriologically con-firmed case of cholera on the Australian mainland occurred when a US air traveller, infected in Bombay, developed cholera after arrival in Melbourne in December 1969. There were two outbreaks of salmonella food poisoning fol-lowing Christmas parties, and an outbreak of diphtheria (indicating that immunisation campaigns were not totally successful). There were also three cases of typhoid, acquired from different sources, emphasising a perpetual epidemic risk. Many severe and complicated cases needing hospital manage-ment, often emergency care and resuscitation, arose from 'routine' epidemics of gastroenteritis, measles, influenza (strain A2 Hong Kong, 1968) and entero-virus disease.

Forbes also commented on an emerging disease hazard that particularly affected Fairfield:

> It is ironical that progress in specific fields of medicine have initiated new epi-demic problems which, stemming from modern general hospitals, pose a unique threat to the community. The increase in hospital-derived Australia antigen (H.A.A.) hepatitis capable of involving the general population in which spread is enhanced particularly by the activities of drug addicts has generated a 'new look' at the need for isolation facilities and care in the prevention of spread of infection [prophetic words]. The increasing use of immunosuppressive drugs and prolonged survival of patients with chronic disease is also providing soil for novel infections.

He also mentioned that consultative services for medical practitioners, other hospitals, health departments in Victoria and interstate, and the Commonwealth Health Department, were extremely time-consuming. For instance, during twelve months, over 3000 telephone inquiries were received from practitioners and other hospitals.

Fairfield's role as a major public health resource for infectious disease information, treatment advice and laboratory testing continued to grow during the following years and eventually superseded patient care as the hospital's main *raison d'être*. In 1971 a new Venereal Diseases Serology Laboratory was established at Fairfield. A nationwide rubella immunisation campaign was

Cholera refers to any one of several intestinal diseases, especially Asiatic cholera, an infection caused by the bacterium *Vibrio-cholerae* and transmitted through contaminated water. Symptoms include violent vomiting and diarrhoea. The disease was first described in India about 400 BCE and is thought to have spread from there. There have been about half a dozen cases of Australia-bound ships carrying the infection—the first recorded was aboard the First Fleet, which reported a case of 'cholera morbus'. Melbourne had two cholera scares in the 1840s, the first in 1841 and the second, reportedly the more serious, in 1849. It is now considered unlikely that those illnesses were in fact cholera. In 1892 two ships were quarantined in Melbourne because of cholera on board, and there have been other such cases.

conducted during the year, marking the beginning of mass immunisation of girls against rubella.

The continuing shortage of trained nursing staff continued to cause 'grave concern', and at times during the year presented serious difficulties in the proper running of the hospital. The hospital considered several proposals for a recruiting campaign, and placed advertisements in various nursing journals in Australia, New Zealand and the United Kingdom. Although the response was not great, some trained staff were obtained by this means.

In the 1970/1971 annual report, Forbes focused on the preventive role and cost-effectiveness of specialised infectious diseases hospitals. As usual, his comments were perceptive and to the point, and are worth quoting at some length:

> The investigation and management of the infectious patients and the impact of epidemic outbreaks endows an integrated Communicable Diseases hospital with a major preventive role in the field of Public Health.
>
> The safe introduction of vaccines and other preventive measures, the search for anonymous agents as well as confirmatory investigation of newly identified agents and the maintenance of various Public Health preventive programs require continual surveillance and with each advance, increasingly specialised technical investigation.
>
> The surveillance and consultative functions and also the central services provided in clinical and laboratory spheres for medical practitioners, other hospitals and the Department of Health contribute to the curtailment of infective disease in the community and in institutions.
>
> The continuing need for patient isolation in this context is emphasised by the impact of serum hepatitis in general hospitals and institutions.
>
> The side-effects of immunisation programs [note the nation-wide rubella immunisation campaign then underway] and related problems impose considerable demands on the consultative functions of this hospital as well as problems of diagnosis and management and information regarding disease prevalence.
>
> The availability of specialised staff and facilities in a modern Communicable Disease hospital for the management of severe and complicated cases and the fluctuating epidemic outbreaks also contribute to reduction of morbidity. The average stay of ten days in 1971 forms a marked contrast with that of more than 30 days in 1939.
>
> Although new and better application of vaccines and perhaps anti-viral agents as well as antibiotics and, indeed, social improvement will achieve further net gains, they also introduce new and novel problems which are occurring through the changing equilibrium in the field of infection. The problems of investigation and management, precise surveillance and continuing re-assessment as a consequence of these changes and also the consequent rise in acceptable standards of medical care will require even more technical investigation in the future.

The central services such as special clinics and laboratory services, e.g. in relation to rubella and Australia antigen problems which have increased so much in recent months, are also factors in the control of community infectious disease.

In addition to the humanitarian aspects of successful control of a number of epidemic diseases such as diphtheria, typhoid, poliomyelitis, rubella, measles and others, the net financial gain to the community, albeit difficult to estimate exactly, is large. Not only must the direct medical cost to the individual and the man hours lost through illness be considered but also factors of family disruption, the restriction of movement by people during major epidemics and, in particular, the financial loss to the community through mortality and chronic disability . . .

The cost of the Communicable or Infectious Disease Centre is dwarfed by the savings resulting from its innate preventive function.

The question of costs or, more accurately, cost/benefit analysis, continued to attract Dr Forbes' attention in 1972. He took the opportunity not only to reflect on the hospital's achievements but also to warn that, if such success was to be maintained, the community would have to be prepared to meet the costs involved in maintaining the hospital as a modern infectious disease facility. It is clear from his argument that he was concerned that the hospital was in danger of being a victim of its own success:

Infective agents and the processes of infection are perpetual ingredients of any society and being adaptive, continue to dominate human activity and consequently, the medical field. It is ironical that public health services which are successful in achieving preventive aims, suffer from the anonymity of 'no news' with the attendant risk of complacency. Not only does the general population lack the stimulus of epidemic threats to ensure immunisation for example, but the administrators of health funds also forget that the price of protection is a continuing one. Expenditure in modern public health programs has suffered in favour of more dramatic fashionable and extremely expensive prestige programs such as cardiac transplantation. Obviously this developing sphere must not be neglected but maintenance of health and treatment of disease in the biologically normal population must retain top priority of concern and research.

The maintenance of a centre with sophisticated facilities based on the concentration of infective patients as a sheet anchor for the establishment of a surveillance organisation, of special clinics and a consulting service performing a central function for the state is an important component in a public health service.

In no field of Medicine have the technical advances been more dramatic and effective than that of communicable diseases in the last 15 years. The quality of modern investigations and treatment of infective diseases continues to introduce new dimensions to routine investigation and management which require continuing revision of facilities if advantage is to be taken of the modern techniques and information available.

During any outbreak, a hospital such as Fairfield must provide facilities to minimise public and newspaper alarm. That this has been achieved successfully with repeated outbreaks should not obscure the recognition of new routine techniques and insufficient modern Wards to provide versatility for the management of patients with infective diseases all of which are acute.

Forbes emphasised that traditional preoccupation with mortality rates was inclined to overshadow the illness and suffering due to infective disease which caused a major community medical problem from both humanitarian and economic viewpoints. He stated that there was no reason for complacency about the dramatically reduced mortalities due to infection, as these were maintained only by continued vigilance and by maintaining progressive specialised standards of patient care and surveillance. On expenses, he noted that:

> As in other spheres the improved performance of a Communicable Diseases Centre such as Fairfield based on new technology may be expected to cost more than in the past. The building program in this hospital has kept pace with modern requirements only by extensive improvisation which has now reached its limits. In the next few years, the increased rate of expenditure on new laboratories and wards will be necessary to keep pace with modern developments and the new standards of hospital practice.

The shortage of trained nursing staff intensified in 1972, causing some restrictions in the admission of patients. The hospital sought 'expert advice' on how best to rectify this increasingly serious problem and, as a result of this advice, a new recruiting program was started. A series of special advertisements, under the title 'Did You Know?', was directed to trained nurses, presenting information regarding the specialised nature of Fairfield hospital. It was hoped that this campaign would ease, if not end, the hospital's shortage of nurses. The success of the measles immunisation campaign was recorded in the 1972 annual report:

> Until 1969, large epidemics of measles have recurred regularly in Melbourne each second year achieving their maximum numbers at the end of the winter. Following a mass immunisation campaign conducted by the Victorian Department of Health during which 202,000 doses of measles vaccine were distributed early in 1971, the admission rates during this year when an epidemic was anticipated, appear to have been modified . . . none of these cases had been immunised.

Fairfield unreservedly welcomed the success of immunisation campaigns such as this, and indeed the hospital had played no small part in promoting the worth of mass immunisation. However, it was becoming increasingly obvious that the consequent dramatic reduction in the prevalence of previously common infectious diseases placed some question marks over the

future role of the hospital. The reduction in threat from 'local' infectious diseases was to some extent counterbalanced by external threats from imported
diseases. This was demonstrated in November 1972, when thirty patients with
cholera were admitted to the hospital; they had been passengers on an aircraft
and had acquired their infection from food taken on in Bahrain.

On a positive note, Fairfield's Nursing Aide School expanded its student
intake in 1972 when students from the Preston and Northcote Community
Hospital and the Royal Melbourne Hospital began attending its courses. The
year also saw major improvements to Wards 6, 15 and 16. On 1 September the
Celsius temperature scale was adopted in place of Fahrenheit—fevers were
quickly reduced, at least mathematically!

The Board endeavoured to speed the upgrading of the facilities. In 1973
it reviewed the outline 'master plan' and also the rebuilding program for the
next four years, and submitted these plans to the Commission of Public
Health and to the Hospitals and Charities Commission. The plans listed major
building works to replace inadequate and out-dated buildings and to provide
for new developments in medicine; other projects involved replacement or
renovation, with relatively small, capital costs, that were considered matters of
urgency from the viewpoint of maintenance and changes of function in the
hospital. After again submitting the 'master plan' (or wish list) for the rebuilding of the hospital, the Board continued intense political lobbying to win
funding for the virology section of the new laboratory. This lobbying was successful, and work began on the new laboratory facility in July 1973.

A description of the hospital and its functions in the 1973 annual report
is of interest because it presents not only a good factual synopsis of the hospital and its functions but also an illuminating insight into how management
viewed the hospital's present and future role:

> The Fairfield Hospital area has been reserved by successive Governments and
> Boards of Management for Public Health purposes relating to infection.
>
> The area contains (1) the hospital and its laboratories which is functioning
> increasingly on a consultative basis through continuous demands as a Com-
> municable Diseases Centre for Victoria and the Commonwealth as well as other
> States and (2) the Exotic Diseases hospital designed primarily as a smallpox hos-
> pital but functioning meantime as a leprosarium available at short notice for its
> primary purpose. The Medical Staff and technical hospital facilities are supplied
> by Fairfield hospital.
>
> The hospital's policy and function contributing to both Health and Hospital
> Services makes its position unique in the Hospital field. Logically, the Hospital
> is established under the Health Act rather than the Hospital Act.

The report commented that Fairfield had evolved as a 'Centre' with
responsibilities and functions beyond primary responsibility of patient care,

and that the notable technical advances in treating and diagnosing infectious diseases (in which the hospital had played a part) had created new technical standards and requirements:

> The more recent continuing technical advances in relation to infective diseases, and the elucidation of many subjects on which information was formerly meagre, have led to greater precision in diagnosis, improvement in management and expansion of the speciality. The changing ecology of viruses in the face of the new patterns of immunity produced by artificial infection with attenuated viruses also requires continuous re-evaluation. The dominant problems and scope of investigation and management now differ extensively from those of the 1940's, 1950's and even 1960's. Enhanced technical capacity has increased the demand for consultation not only on the individual level but also at national and international levels.

Patients at Fairfield needed specialised facilities for varied conditions, for example, facilities for infants with croup, artificial respiration for patients with respiratory paralysis, haemodialysis for infective patients with renal failure, particularly those with hepatitis B unsafe for the general dialysis units and 'special care' facilities for the management of all types of life-threatening infections from meningitis to septicaemic shock:

> These facilities and staff cannot be instituted on a fragmented basis in a multi-plicity of small units which would have insufficient material to generate exper-tise nor would there be sufficient staff which is required on a whole-time basis.
>   In addition, the communicable Diseases Hospital is required in a large popu-lation to meet rapidly fluctuating epidemic demands which cannot be met at General Hospitals without gross disruption of their function.

The Interim Hospitals and Health Services Commission, chaired by Dr Sidney Sax, was established on 19 December 1973. The year also saw the hos-pital's Matron, Vivian Bullwinkel, receive the MBE in the New Year's Honours List—an award that gave great pleasure to the whole Fairfield com-munity. Dr A. Kucers, a specialist physician at the hospital, published a medi-cal textbook entitled *The Use of Antibiotics*. It was favourably reviewed in the prestigious medical journals the *Lancet* and the *British Medical Journal*, and its reception in the international medical community brought considerable reflected glory to the hospital.

Sir Albert Coates KtB, OBE, MD, MS, Hon. LLD, FRCS, FRACS, who had been chair of the Board since 1956, informed the Board in July 1973 that he intended to retire from the position. Sir Albert remained a member of the Board until his death in 1977.

The Board noted that the resources of the hospital had been heavily taxed during 1974. The two major problems 'continued to be the shortage of trained Nursing Staff, and the replacement of inadequate and out-dated buildings'.

In the 1974 annual report Dr Forbes noted that the hospital had been asked to comment on the requirements of a Regional Medical Centre in a rural city for the management of infectious diseases; this prompted him to describe the function of the hospital in the context of state requirements:

> Such Hospitals [as Fairfield] form a part of the Public Health Service as distinct from a Hospital Service per se ... An important function of the central infectious diseases hospital is maintenance of reserve beds for the frequent epidemic emergencies, a continuing requirement in a large urban population, and also to provide for epidemic overflows from regional centres as well as the admission of patients who require special investigation and care, exemplified this year during the outbreak of Murray Valley Encephalitis, [twenty two patients were admitted to Fairfield].
>
> All Communicable and Infectious Diseases Units irrespective of size must be administered predominantly as consultant inpatient centres having patients referred from their homes or other Hospitals by telephone so that they may be admitted directly to an isolation ward or area to avert the certainty of cross infection in a hospital outpatients department or reception area.
>
> Suspected cases and particularly patients with undiagnosed fevers must be managed in isolation ... Close liaison with the Public Health Service in the field of infectious disease is essential to extend the surveillance innate in patient care into the allied province of preventive medicine.

The outbreak of Murray Valley encephalitis, while obviously to be deplored, nonetheless gave Dr Forbes the opportunity to use his expertise and experience to investigate a fairly 'exotic' infectious disease. That it was an opportunity he relished can be seen in his report on the outbreak, which not only describes Murray Valley encephalitis but also contains some inspired detective work which resulted in a significant contribution to the under-standing of the aetiology of the virus:

> The onset of the epidemic became apparent with the admission to this Hospital of three patients from the region of the Murray River with severe encephalitis during the second week of January. Subsequently nineteen more patients were managed here during the course of the epidemic [four of the patients admitted to Fairfield with M.V.E. died in the Hospital as a result of the disease giving a fatality rate of 18.18per cent] ... The first twenty recognised human cases were restricted to the Murray River region until the tenth week of the epi-demic when, on February 19, about seven weeks after the first case, symptoms developed in a baby in Windorah in Queensland.

Fourteen cases emerged in Queensland and the Northern Territories in the next nine weeks and one in the north-east of Western Australia, along with a further 24 in the Murray River region. The epidemic therefore covered six states, but was most severe in northern Victoria. Dr Forbes noted that:

> All patients diagnosed as Murray Valley Encephalitis had impairment of cerebral function as distinct from meningitis. Some of the severe cases in addition to gross cerebral dysfunction and coma also developed upper and lower motor neurone paralysis . . . Serological surveys indicated that 37 per cent of the adult population in the Mildura district (Total approximately 30,000) were infected during the outbreak without developing symptoms along with the occurrence of 6 cases of encephalitis. This conformed with other areas further up the River Murray where the infection rates progressively diminished . . .

It is interesting to note that evidence suggests that the virus is endemic in northern Queensland, but epidemics became apparent in the populated areas of the Murray Valley proper and in northern Victoria.

Water birds appear to be the primary reservoir of infection for the virus (as they are for Japanese B encephalitis). The mosquito, *Culex annulirostris,* appears to be the main vector of spread to other species, including humans. It was suggested in 1952 that outbreaks of Murray Valley encephalitis might be a sequel to heavy rain in eastern Australia, in the Darling River catchment area or in the vicinity of the Gulf of Carpentaria in the preceding spring months, extending favourable areas for inland water birds. However, Forbes commented that:

> although the epidemics have been preceded by high rainfall in the Darling catchment, since 1914 these conditions have prevailed on 19 occasions but have been followed by epidemics in only seven of these years and in only 4 did the virus reach the Murray River region, so that additional features must be sought. Examination of the geographical map of Australia reveals four main watersheds in central-eastern Australia which encompass numerous Rainfall Areas from which records have been compiled for over 100 years . . . In ordinary seasons higher rainfall areas in the north and the south are separated by a large semi-arid region . . . Cases occurred in the vicinity of the Murray River in 1918, 1951, 1956 and 1974 but [not] in 1917 when Queensland [and] Northern NSW down to Broken Hill were the main areas, nor in 1922 when the epidemic appeared to be confined mainly to Queensland and 1925 when a similar pattern to that of 1917 recurred. In the years of the large epidemics involving the Murray River Valley proper in 1918, 1951 and 1974, rainfall was excessive in one or both quarters of the previous summers of 1916–17, 1949–50 and 1973–74 in all four of the main watersheds. . . In the other years 1917, 1922 and 1925 when cases were confined to Queensland and New South Wales, the pluvial pattern though present in the northern three catchments, was absent in the Lachlan Murrumbidgee Murray Area.

He concluded that 'two successive wet seasons are required to establish conditions favouring the prolific breeding of water birds and the establishment of a reservoir of virus in northern areas'.

Research work on infectious diseases at Fairfield was by no means limited to 'local' infectious diseases or to the specialities and interests of medical staff. As part of the world scientific community the hospital was involved in a number of major collaborative studies under the auspices of the World Health Organisation. There were five projects in 1974:

- phase 2 of the hepatitis B study defining the carrier rate of Hepatitis B antigen in the general population (giving an indication of exposure to hepatitis B virus);
- phase 2 of the collaborative study to determine the frequency and time of acquisition of cytomegalovirus antibody in the first four years of life (cytomegalovirus is a herpes virus);
- a study involving the use of radial-immuno diffusion to detect antibodies to Influenza A virus;
- study on the association of central nervous system disease with viral infections other than enteroviruses and mumps virus;
- producing a large volume of respiratory syncytial virus complement fixing antigen to be used as a reference reagent.

The importance of the role the hospital played in the international medical community was highlighted when Dr Ian Gust, Fairfield's Medical Virologist, was invited by the World Health Organisation to serve for five years as a member of the Expert Advisory Panel on Virus Diseases. The excellent work being undertaken by Gust and his co-workers was given a boost when a new Microbiology Laboratory (under Gust) was officially opened by Alan Scanlan, Minister for Health, on 20 August 1975. The laboratory was described as 'one of the most modern of its kind in South-East Asia'.

That year was one of the most dramatic not only in Australian political history but also, albeit on a somewhat smaller scale, in the history of Fairfield. As a number of staff, including Dr John Forbes, had already spent time in medical missions to war-torn Vietnam it was hardly surprising that, in the emergency created by the death throes of that long war, the Commonwealth government turned to Fairfield for assistance. Even when describing these dramatic events, Forbes did not neglect to promote the importance of maintaining Fairfield as a specialised infectious disease facility:

> Versatility is an essential feature of the specialised Communicable Diseases Hospital which must necessarily provide space and facilities for large numbers of patients at short notice. A General Hospital consisting as it does of a complex

of specialities cannot provide facilities without disrupting the general function-ing of the Medical Services for which it is designed.

Whilst epidemics and quarantine emergencies usually create the demands, the evacuation by air of waifs from Vietnam in April 1975 provided analogous problems in that with a short period of warning, facilities were available for the admission of babies and children with a variety of diseases, mainly infective and most of them requiring management in Hospital, some intensive care.

The world is shrinking by virtue of efficient communications and rapid transport so that similar problems are likely to recur in various guises including the quarantine screening and treatment of refugees, the necessity for which has been most apparent in groups from Timor which, without medical clearances, have presented a continuing train of infective problems which were predictable but not treated on arrival.

Forbes pointed out that the evacuation of orphans from Vietnam in April 1975 differed from most quarantine situations. The Commonwealth govern-ment had requested that nurses and doctors be made available to proceed to Saigon to receive and transport by air an unknown number of babies and children, many of whom were ill with bowel infections and other unspecified illnesses. Only seventeen hours warning was provided before the outward flight. (The last US personnel in South Vietnam were evacuated by helicopter from the Saigon Embassy compound on 29 April). Clinical staff experienced in the management of acute infective disease in babies and young children were provided by Fairfield and the Repatriation Department, providing the balance of the nurses for management during transportation. Doctors from the Quarantine Section travelled on the aircraft to fulfil immunisation requirements.

After one cancellation (ordered by the federal government) the oper-ation proceeded a week later. The 73 evacuees were fewer than anticipated as many had died during the week's delay. A Boeing 707 flew to and from Bangkok, where the medical group and nurses transhipped to RAAF Hercules aircraft to collect the evacuees from the airport at Saigon. Some preliminary assessment and care was possible in the flight from Saigon to Bangkok, where the evacuees were transferred to the Boeing aircraft, a section of which had been set aside for resuscitation and treatment of those with severe symptoms. Shortly after leaving Saigon, one infant died as a result of dehydration due to a bowel infection. Many were seriously ill:

> 22 (30%) of the children were found to have various grades of recognisable mal-nutrition and 19 of these were anaemic. Persistent devoted nursing was required to establish suitable programs for the very small babies . . . About 50% of the children had some skin infection, either impetigo or skin or scalp abscesses. Eight children had gastro-enteritis. Bacterial bowel pathogens were isolated

from 9 (14%) of the children; 8 strains of Salmonellae (4 untyped, 2 havana, 1 seftenberg, 1 lexington) and two Shigella strains (1 sonne, 1 flexneri Type 1) . . . Hepatitis B virus was detected in the blood of 14 (19%) children [over] three months. Three of these children [had] current hepatitis. Fourteen children had ear infections and three conjunctivitis. Six had oral thrush, two developed varicella and another developed whooping cough. One child had congenital syphilis with bony and meningeal involvement . . . Five children died: three failed to thrive due to gastro-enteritis . . . and two malnourished babies died as a result of pneumocystis carinii pneumonia, which developed acutely 9 weeks after admission . . .

The long and somewhat fearfully awaited *Report of the Committee of Inquiry into Hospital and Health Services in Victoria* was published in 1976. In reference to Fairfield the report concluded:

(i)   We think that the policy of centralising infectious diseases treatment at Fairfield Hospital is a sound one, and that the diseases of this nature, particularly those that occur only rarely or periodically, a dispersal of expertise is to be avoided;
(ii) An Epidemiological Section is required to research disease incidence and to operate as an effective preventive measure. This could be located at Fairfield where infectious disease beds as well as laboratory facilities are available.[2]

Fairfield extended its role as a central infectious disease facility by initiating meetings to pave the way for the formation of a national infectious diseases society. Forbes (who had received the Order of Australia during the year) in the 1976 annual report once again reflected on the role of the hospital. The fact that the Medical Superintendent felt it necessary to constantly justify the existence of a specialised infectious diseases hospital shows how constant the threat to the hospital's future was. Fairfield's future was never *secure*: even in 'good' years there was a perceived threat to its future. Forbes had this to say:

An infectious diseases hospital with an integrated specialised laboratory has great natural potential as a Centre for Disease Control. The laboratory service, whose function is integrated with clinical aspects, thrives with the stimulus of patients care and the combined approach yields more complete information.

By virtue of the facilities which have evolved to meet the demands imposed by the new technical advances in patient care and investigation particularly in virology and in the epidemiological extensions of these, the mantle of a communicable disease centre has fallen on this hospital almost involuntarily.

Apart from managing the severe and complicated common infectious diseases, providing continuity of experience in the management of the now intermittent vaccine-controlled diseases such as diphtheria and poliomyelitis and the investigation of unknown fevers and outbreaks, involvement with overseas problems is a feature of its capability.

The increasing demands in this field are reflected in the admission rates of malaria, 4 cases in 1961 steadily increasing to 44 cases in 1975.

With strong Public Health affiliations, the provision of a surveillance service is axiomatic and the investigation and management of quarantinable diseases including the more exotic complaints is a natural function when these problems arise.

Forbes emphasised that Fairfield required 'special care' provisions for life-threatening infections, facilities for artificial respiration and the management of croup and, with the advent of hepatitis B, haemodialysis equipment, as well as facilities for safe isolation of patients. At that time, smallpox was still a threat, and horrific new diseases such as lassa fever had emerged. Air travel, which was becoming more common, increased the risk of importing exotic diseases still in the incubation stage. Thus provision of high security ward and laboratory facilities was essential:

> The abrupt demand for facilities to isolate and manage a large number of cases of cholera in 1972 emphasise the reality of the quarantine problems. The known case or contact constitutes a tangible risk situation, but the increasing number of patients returning from overseas areas with fevers unidentified at the time of admission to hospital, form the main problem which requires specialised awareness, current information derived from sources such as W.H.O. and C.D.C. in the United States, and at this stage, re-examination of isolation requirements.
>
> Facilities and techniques for managing such a patient should automatically obviate any risk to other patients and staff not in contact with the patients and present a minimum risk to staff caring for that patient. To achieve this, facilities must be provided for the admission of all patients individually in rooms designed to obviate any risk of the spread of infection including exotic airborne agents which necessitates the provision of a high-security air handling system in a proportion of the cubicles. For certain types of exotic infection, air effluent and wastes must be made safe at points of exit. The concepts are by no means unique but their design must necessarily be meticulous. The realization that such facilities become effective only through the constant practice by staff of appropriate isolation techniques is vital.

Melbourne had a Lassa fever scare in 1976. Lassa fever, a haemorrhagic fever originating in Lassa, Nigeria, and apparently first spread by mouse urine, had entered the public imagination—rightly or wrongly—as one of the great infectious disease fears of the decade. The incident occurred when an 87-year-old Australian man visiting Britain was admitted to hospital in London with a blocked artery. As luck would have it, he was treated in a ward containing a patient later discovered to be suffering from Lassa fever. On his

return to Australia, and before the Lassa fever contact in London was diagnosed and British public health authorities advised Australian authorities
about the risk, the man was admitted to a ward alongside four other patients
in Box Hill hospital. The five at-risk contacts were transferred from Box Hill
Hospital to the Exotic Diseases Unit at Fairfield, and blood samples were sent
to the high-security laboratory at the Centre for Disease Control in Atlanta,
Georgia. Fortunately these tests proved negative, and the risk of an outbreak
of this virulent and deadly virus in Australia passed.

It is fortunate indeed that the man concerned had not been infected by
the virus. As Sandland noted in his history of Fairfield, 'For such a disease the
existing arrangements for protecting staff from contracting the disease or
spreading it would be quite inadequate, hence the planned High Security
Quarantine Unit to be included soon, as an addition to Fairfield's facilities'.[3]

Among interesting developments during 1976 were the Board's acceptance of an invitation, through the Richmond Herald of Arms in London, to
obtain an official grant of the hospital coat of arms. And, following the successful rehabilitation of a patient who became blind, the hospital produced a
short educational film, in conjunction with the Guide Dogs Association, on
the rehabilitation of blind patients.

Although no one at Fairfield, or indeed anywhere else in the world, was
aware of the significance of the event, the death of two homosexual men
in San Francisco from Kaposi's sarcoma in 1977 is now thought to herald
the onset of one of the most deadly viruses and most tragic epidemics in
human history—acquired immune deficiency syndrome / human immunodeficiency virus (HIV/AIDS). It was to be some years before Fairfield would
be called to treat HIV/AIDS patients.

The year also saw the resignation of Matron Vivian Bullwinkel MBE,
ARRC, FMN, DipN (Aust), FCNA, ED. Bullwinkel, one of the most famous
nurses in Australian history, had been Matron since 1961 and had served the
hospital, the nursing profession and her country with great distinction. A sign
of the still sexist times is that an annual report shortly after her retirement
noted that she had 'resigned to become Mrs. Frank Statham and live in
Perth'. The Board held a farewell dinner in Matron Bullwinkel's honour on
23 November 1977.

Margaret Lafferty, who had been Deputy Matron since 1974, was
appointed Director of Nursing on Matron Bullwinkel's resignation. Two
other notable resignations at this time were those of Victor I. Frank, who
had served the hospital as Chief Pharmacist for twenty-nine years, and
G. McKenzie, who had been Stores Officer for twenty-six years. Too often
the ancillary and administrative staff who are essential to the running of

Sister Vivian Bullwinkel was born on 18 December 1915 at Kapunda in South Australia, educated at Broken Hill High School and completed nursing training at Broken Hill Hospital.

She enlisted in the Australian Army Nursing Service at the start of World War II and was posted to Malaya in 1941. She was the sole survivor of a massacre of twenty-two Australian nurses and a boatload of British troops by Japanese soldiers on the beach on Bangka Island in 1942. Her ship, the *Vyner Brooke*, when escaping from Singapore with some three hundred passengers, including sixty-five nurses, had been bombed and sunk with great loss of life in the Bangka Straits. After hiding in the jungle for ten days she was recaptured and endured extraordinarily harsh conditions as a prisoner of war for the next three years.

Widely acclaimed for her heroism when she returned to Australia after the war, she was awarded the Florence Nightingale Medal in 1947. She gave evidence at the International Military Tribunal in Tokyo. Elizabeth Burchill in her study of *Australian Nurses Since Nightingale 1860–1990* describes Bullwinkel as the 'most famous and highly decorated nurse of the Second World War'.

After the war she became very prominent in Australian nursing, being appointed matron of Fairfield Hospital in 1961 and serving the hospital with great distinction until 1977. She became the first female trustee of the Australian War Memorial in 1971.

hospitals are not given sufficient credit for the contributions that they make, and we should always be aware of the many and varied jobs that need to be done if a hospital is to function effectively and efficiently. Although the years of service of Frank and McKenzie were notable—and by today's standards exceptional—by the standards of the time such long service, such commitment, was not uncommon. Many staff at Fairfield served the hospital for decade after decade, often for little financial recompense or recognition.

While discussing faithful service to the hospital over many years, it is appropriate to note that the Fairfield Hospital Auxiliary, which had operated for over thirty years, ceased to function due to lack of members in 1977. The voluntary workers of the Auxiliary had supported the hospital in a multitude of tangible and intangible ways, and the patients and staff had good cause to mourn the passing of such a staunch friend.

The first annual meeting of the Australasian Society for Infectious Diseases was held in Melbourne in March 1977. This society originated at Fairfield, and much of the credit for its formation is due to Dr John Forbes, its foundation president, and Sir Macfarlane Burnet, its patron. An annual address was named in Macfarlane Burnet's honour.

Two old enemies of society in general and Fairfield in particular forced their way back onto the agenda during 1977. A serious typhoid outbreak at Eastland Shopping Centre, which led to 127 admissions, 37 of whom were found to have the disease, reminding the community that by no means all the

Dr John A. Forbes was Medical Superintendent of Fairfield from 1 January 1961 to 31 December 1978, and prior to that was Senior Medical Officer in 1953 and Deputy Medical Superintendent from 1954 to 1960. As Medical Superintendent, he ensured continuation of the highest standards of medical and nursing services at Fairfield, and helped to maintain the hospital's status as a world leader. He made a major contribution to public health services and, as the spokesman for Fairfield, consistently received wide and favourable support from the news media. Because of his high standing within his profession, Forbes did much to preserve and develop the role of Fairfield as a communicable diseases centre.

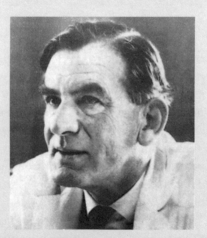

Dr John Forbes, Medical Superintendent 1961–1978.

dreaded infectious diseases that had blighted the lives of our forebears had been eradicated. More positively, in February 1977 Dr N. Bennett joined the International Commission on the Eradication of Smallpox in Pakistan and Afghanistan at the invitation of the World Health Organisation. Bennett's participation in this important international commission reflected well on the international standing of the hospital and its staff.

Important new equipment was acquired during the year. Carlton and United Breweries Ltd agreed to donate a replacement ambulance for use by poliomyelitis patients. This specially equipped vehicle enabled patients to go on outings and greatly improved to their independence and consequently their quality of life. The hospital also acquired Carba Linguaduc patient-operated electronic equipment for use during occupational therapy sessions. This comprised a typewriter and several page-turners which could be operated by otherwise totally dependent patients. The staff reported that it had been 'enthusiastically accepted by our long-term patients, as it provides them with a considerable degree of independence for personal reading and correspondence'.

A condensed history of the hospital presented in the 1979 annual report to mark the seventy-fifth anniversary of the hospital recorded the two perennial problems:

> In the mid-1970s the hospital had two big problems, a shortage of trained nursing staff and the continued failure of the hospital to receive funding for a rebuilding program. One undoubted factor related to the rebuilding inertia was that the hospital was completely funded by the Government and, therefore, had no private funds and was unable to mount public appeals. Although permission for a new Nurse Teaching Unit and a Clinical Services Block and Ward were obtained in 1976, the former was delayed until 1978 and for a variety of reasons, the latter have yet to eventuate.

Sadly, 1978 brought the resignation of Medical Superintendent Dr John Forbes, AM, MB, BS, FRACP, FACMA. Forbes had been associated with the hospital for over a quarter of a century and had been Medical Superintendent since 1961. Not the least of his contributions to the treatment and care of infectious disease was his tireless promotion of the medical speciality of infectious disease medicine and his commitment to training young infectious disease physicians at Fairfield. In his final report Forbes took the opportunity to review the field of infectious disease management:

> The optimism engendered in the early 1950's by the decline of diphtheria, the availability of penicillin to treat streptococcal infections and the reduction of deaths due to whooping cough which led to the catch-cry that infectious diseases were finished was ill-informed. It is true that these scourges had

dominated the health scene particularly amongst children and the admitting policy of the hospital had been conditioned accordingly. Little was known of the multitude of viruses which are now household words and the dynamic equilibrium basic to the epidemiology of infective agents particularly viruses and their inter-dependence on social conditions.

Standards of health care and results of treatment changed, so that what appeared previously to be tolerable morbidity and mortality figures due to the common diseases of childhood became unacceptable without those of diphtheria, scarlet fever and whooping cough to dwarf them. The mortality from infectious diseases fell during this period, but the morbidity remained high, particularly with the emergence of additional epidemic problems such as hepatitis and enterovirus disease. Despite the control of diphtheria, whooping cough and tetanus, poliomyelitis which had emerged as a major epidemic problem in 1937 recurred in epidemic form each year from 1946 to 1956 when Salk and later Sabin vaccine provided respite.

The development by Dr John Enders of tissue culture as a medium for the routine identification and cultivation of polio virus and later many other virus types, revitalised a speciality in which precise knowledge of one major facet, namely, the viruses, had been unknowingly meagre. Survey work using Enders' technique revealed the genesis of a large group of epidemic virus diseases which were emerging with improved standards of living and infant hygiene, so that primary infection was occurring in older age groups. Poliomyelitis was the first of these appearing as a major epidemic in 1937 and in 1953 hepatitis A emerged as an overt epidemic problem, whilst the various enteroviruses have become annual epidemic agents.

The changing admission policy demanded by the changing patterns of disease produced a considerably different spectrum of infectious disease requiring hospital care. Previously anonymous agents were identified and the formerly ill-segregated symptomatology of diseases such as bronchiolitis in babies were defined. The viruses causing the common diseases of childhood were identified in laboratory culture and vaccines also became available during the 1960's for measles, rubella and mumps . . . Gastro-enteritis became more dominant in the spectrum of disease over the period and in recent years the identification of rotavirus has partially, but only partially, filled the identification gap which still remains a challenge. The mortalities and stay in hospital too are vastly different, but certain of the viral diseases still await the development of effective anti-viral agents.

Whooping cough is one disease which has retained its cyclical epidemic pattern throughout the period, but with a notable reduction in mortality and complications mainly through the successful treatment of the secondary infections and atelectatic phenomena. The epidemics which occur each 3–4 years develop slowly, reach their peak after twelve months or so, and subside gradually. Whilst vaccine breakthroughs are recorded in these reports, there is little doubt that the disease is ameliorated by vaccine with greatly reduced numbers with characteristic pertussis. Success in other medical fields with the prolongation of life of subjects with conditions such as leukemia which are associated with immunological deficiencies have introduced previously uncommon idiosyncratic problems of infection.

Most patients for whom admission was sought were suffering from severe and complicated common infectious diseases, could not be managed at home, and their admission to a general hospital was inadvisable. The pandemic of Asian A strain of influenza in 1957 emphasised the value of an epidemic hospital in a large modern city.

The increasing availability and popularity of air travel was increasing the danger of importing exotic diseases. In the 1950s, tropical disease was a rare reason for admission but, with a large travelling population, this became a steadily increasing problem—as shown particularly by the numbers of patients admitted with malaria. Managing quarantine problems and investigating returning travellers with mysterious illnesses was always a function of Fairfield. Immigrants and refugees could also bring with them diseases non-endemic to Australia. Although, for example, smallpox was no longer a major world problem, the emergence of the African haemorrhagic fevers created a greater need for high security nursing and laboratory facilities.

Following Dr Forbes' resignation came the retirement of Manager and Secretary, Basil D. Dynon:

> Mr. Dynon remained at the hospital until February 1979, thereby completing nearly 46 years of service, being Manager and Secretary for a record period of 28 years. He carried out his role as Executive Officer of the hospital and Secretary of the Board in a quiet efficient manner. He was always fair in his decisions and performed numerous deeds of kindness, the source of which were often unknown to the recipients. He was a trusted adviser to the Board and a confidant of all the many Chairmen of the Board with whom he worked. He never used his position for any personal gain. Undoubtedly, his loyal support of successive Medical Superintendents was a great factor in ensuring the internal strength of the hospital. To this day, Bas is very active and maintains a keen interest in the hospital and its welfare.

The Board recorded the following minute of appreciation:

> The Board of Management of Fairfield Hospital expresses to Mr. Basil D. Dynon F.C.I.S., A.A.S.A. (Sen.), its warmest thanks for his services to the hospital as a member of the administrative staff from 30th June, 1933, to 29th August, 1950, and as Manager and Secretary from 31st May, 1950, to 16th February, 1979. During his long period of service, Mr Dynon has seen many changes in the hospital, its staff, and in the Board itself, and in all these situations he has consistently given loyal and outstanding service. His competence in general administration, and his ability to obtain the co-operation of those who have

served under, and with him, have contributed much to the successful functioning and growth of the hospital. In particular the Board Members have learned to appreciate his guidance and help. The Board records appreciation of his long and faithful service, and wishes him a happy and rewarding retirement.

The year also saw the opening of the Vivian Bullwinkel School of Nursing. Bullwinkel returned to the hospital for the opening of the unit named in her honour. The building was designed by architect Stewart, Pinniger, who designed all Fairfield buildings until his death in August 1979.

Malaria is one of today's most serious health problems. The disease is now mainly confined to areas of Africa, Asia and Latin America, where millions of people are affected. The symptoms (periodic attacks of fever, shivering, chills, pain in the joints and headache) have been known for hundreds of years, though the cause was not established until the late nineteenth century. In the fifth century BCE, Hippocrates differentiated three types of malarial fever, according to the timing of recurring bouts, and noted a connection between malaria and proximity to stagnant water.

It was thought that 'miasma' (*'mal aria'* means 'bad air' in Italian) from swamps caused the disease, until Alphonse Laveran in 1880 found that malaria was caused by protozoans. Towards the end of the nineteenth century it was established that these parasites were transmitted to humans by the bites of female Anopheline mosquitoes. Four species of Plasmodium can produce the disease in its various forms— *Plasmodium falciparum* (the most widespread and dangerous),. *Plasmodium vivax, Plasmodium ovale* and *Plasmodium malaria*. Treatment of the symptoms were in use long before the cause was known. Infusions of *qinghao* (*Artemisia annua*) has been used in China for at least two thousand years; its active ingredient, *qinghaosu* (artemisinin) has recently been identified. In Peru the bitter bark of the cinchona tree (*Cinchona ledgeriana*) was used to treat malarial fever well before the fifteenth century. The most active compound of cinchona bark, quinine, which has been used to treat millions of malaria sufferers, was isolated in 1820. In the 1940s drugs such as chloroquine, paraquine, pyrimethamine and amodiaquin were synthesised. Research into developing vaccines is being undertaken in many countries, including Australia.

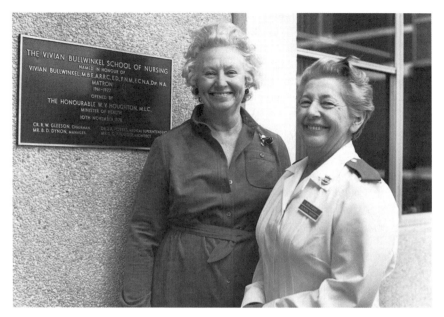

Sister Vivian Bullwinkel (left) and Sister Shirley Boden at the opening of the Sister Vivian Bullwinkel School of Nursing in November 1978.

After lengthy discussions between Fairfield and the Commonwealth Department of Health, the government decided to build a national High-Security Quarantine Unit at Fairfield. This was a response to the increasing danger posed by imported viral haemorrhagic fevers (the Lassa fever scare three years before may have helped to expedite this move). Wards 9 and 10 were demolished in September 1978 to make room for the new quarantine ward, but the site was later changed to an area north of the exotic diseases hospital. The speed with which infectious diseases could be spread in the modern global village, and the need for a high security quarantine unit, were highlighted by the widespread publicity and public disquiet relating to international cholera transmission via aircraft travel. Construction commenced on the quarantine unit in 1979.

Towards the end of the year the hospital was the scene of a serious breach of security when a dangerous prisoner who had been receiving treatment contrived to escape. While the escape had its serious side, the Keystone Cops quality of the events added a farcical element:

> Convicted double murderer Barry Robert Quinn—described by police as one of Australia's most dangerous criminals—may seek medical treatment in the next few days.

Quinn, 31, escaped from the Fairfield Infectious Diseases hospital, where he was being treated for hepatitis, on Thursday night ... Sergeant Ritchie said Quinn was extremely dangerous and should not be confronted by anyone who recognised him ... Quinn was serving a life sentence in Pentridge for the murder of two men at the Car-O-Tel Motel in St Kilda four years ago.

He escaped at 7.40 by jumping through an unbarred window and running to a waiting car which was parked around a corner near the hospital.

The Chief of the CIB (Administration), Detective Chief Superintendent Eric Janatzki, said yesterday a get-well card posted in the city on Sunday was apparently the signal for the escape's go-ahead.

The card contained the message: 'Barry, here's hoping healthier happier days are just around the corner.'

Detectives are still examining the card for any more clues to the escape.

Police said Quinn, who was in an isolation ward at the Fairfield Hospital, was visited each day by a young woman.

But two prison officers assigned to guard were not allowed to stay in the room with him. They had to watch through an open door.

Police said when the woman visited Quinn on Thursday she drew a curtain around the bed and later left saying she was going for some cigarettes. When she failed to return guards searched the room and found Quinn had escaped.

Police said he is about 170 centimetres tall, with fair complexion, blue eyes and a slight to medium build. He has a small star tattooed on each cheek ... The Social Welfare Minister, Mr Dixon, admitted last night that Fairfield Hospital's security arrangements were seriously inadequate.

He said that security guidelines would be reviewed for all prisoner visits to the hospital, following Thursday's escape. [4]

With the 'Old Guard'—Bullwinkel, Forbes and Dynon—departing the scene, the Board instituted a major restructuring of the administration of the hospital. Reflecting the growing 'cult' of managerialism, we can with hindsight see that this decision was to play a large part in the extraordinarily turbulent and divisive years which followed. Dr Noel McKenzie Bennett was appointed to the dual positions of Chief Executive Officer and Medical Director, with Graeme Houghton as Director of Administrative Services and Dr Alvis Kucers as Physician in Charge of Medical Services.

The 1979 annual report contained some fascinating reflections on its history, personalities, and future:

Historical comparisons:
Although the annual admission rate has again had a slight fall, the diversity of diseases treated is greater than ever before. For example, in 1955 about 20 principal infectious diseases were recorded in the annual report, but today this number has more than trebled. As a result of increasing travel by Australians, the hospital now functions as a centre for the treatment of tropical diseases. This role

has been recently emphasised by the influx of refugees from Vietnam who not only bring diseases which are non-endemic to our community but they may well lead to a recrudescence of older diseases such as tuberculosis. Factors influencing the recent fall in the demand for beds for patients with infections are the reduced birth rate in the community and the recent absence of large epidemics. A glance at the annual admission numbers since 1915 reveals that a cyclical variation in the numbers of patients with infectious diseases has been a characteristic of our community. The policies enunciated in 1956 that the function of the hospital must be preserved and it must remain prepared to cope with unexpected epidemics are just as timely in 1979. Fairfield Hospital today not only serves the State of Victoria but also the whole of Australia. The laboratory is continually being recognised as an expanding reference centre. In addition, the formation of an Air Medical Evacuation Team at the hospital to bring high risk patients to the special High Security Quarantine Ward at the hospital from all over Australia, reflects our important national function.

Personalities:

The Hospital is a large organisation and over a period of 25 years many personnel come and go. It is very difficult to single out other personalities, but the names of longstanding medical consultants Dr Stanley Williams, Sir Ian Wood, Dr Gordon Donnan, Mr. Ian Heinz, Dr John Billings, Dr Bernard Gilligan, Dr James Bottcher, Dr Max Robinson, Dr Tom Hurley, Dr Brian Fargher and Dr Frank Forster well deserve recording. Mr. Harry George, the predecessor to our present engineer, Mr. Neil McDonald who was appointed in 1969, was a perfectionist who kept an 'old machine' functioning well. There were many devoted members of the nursing and administrative staff who contributed in so many different ways to the success of the hospital. Some of these are Sisters Scott, Ferguson, Cogan and Robinson and Messrs. Jack Goujon, 'Mac' Colwell and Bill McGennisken. For the sake of brevity the legion of Fairfield friends and staff must remain anonymous.

The Future:

[Fairfield] fulfils its role in infectious diseases at a standard comparable with any similar institute in the world. Tested facilities and staff are available to cope with unexpected epidemics or outbreaks of disease. Resources for the microbiological investigation of infectious diseases are probably equal to any in the world. In the care of patients with infectious diseases, the use of antibiotics and microbiological research, our medical staff are internationally recognised experts. By the establishment of the High Security Quarantine Ward at Fairfield Hospital, the Commonwealth has given due cognisance to the specialised resources of the hospital. Nevertheless, the present standards at the Hospital cannot be maintained unless the present buildings are progressively renovated and rebuilt ... The newly formed Health Commission of Victoria is at present in its planning phase and is committed to a rationalisation of present health services ... it is hoped the overall development and rebuilding of the Hospital can be co-ordinated with the Public Health needs of the State. It is possible that by the turn of the century, the Fairfield Hospital campus will be converted into a large integrated Public Health Centre incorporating and supporting the functions of the Hospital.

But then again, perhaps not.

Following a request by the Health Commission, an overflow of patients with tuberculosis from Heatherton Sanatorium was accepted into Fairfield in February 1979. This resulted from an increased demand for beds for patients with tuberculosis, particularly Vietnamese refugees. After another request from the Health Commission, the Board of Management later accepted transfer of the control of the adjacent Exotic Diseases Hospital, and the responsibility for providing institutional care for patients with Hansen's disease, from 30 June. In his first report as Chief Executive Officer Dr Bennett said:

> The first Annual Report of the Hospital was published in 1915, and contained a Medical Superintendent's Report detailing the principal diseases admitted during the year and the results of treatment. In all succeeding reports, these statistics were repeated and gradually expanded until the present format was established. In times of escalating hospital costs and when means of assessing the efficiency of health care are being sought, the statistics recorded in the Annual Report of Fairfield Hospital are unique in Australia. By virtue of its specialised function, Fairfield Hospital Reports also provide an invaluable historical record of the incidence of infectious diseases in the State of Victoria spanning a period of 65 years.

Dr Bennet also took the opportunity to describe the background and operations of the proposed quarantine facility to be based at Fairfield:

> The Hospital's New Role in Quarantinable Diseases. In the last 12 years, three new viral diseases have originated in Africa, Marburg virus disease (1967), Lassa fever (1969) and Ebola virus disease (1976). In certain circumstances, these diseases have been highly infectious and have had a high mortality. Both Marburg virus disease and Lassa fever have been imported into developed countries. As a result, many nations have evolved plans to cope with the possible importation of these diseases; Australia has been amongst the foremost of these.
>
> In 1975, Lassa fever and Marburg virus disease were proclaimed as quarantinable diseases. In 1977, it was decided that quarantine stations that had been constructed in the last century or earlier in this century, primarily to isolate patients with smallpox, were unsuitable for these new virus diseases. They were often old, often remote from specialised treatment and not capable of providing 'high security'.
>
> The Commonwealth Department of Health recommended that a national high security unit should be built at Fairfield Hospital and that present quarantine stations should be progressively closed. In 1978, the Board of Management of Fairfield Hospital and the Health Commission of Victoria approved the

building of this unit; construction will begin in the second half of 1979 and be completed in 1980.

Patients suspected of having one of these African fevers will be transferred to this special unit at the discretion of the Medical Officer appointed for this purpose in each state. A suspect patient will be placed in a special transit isolator and transported by a specially chartered aircraft to Fairfield Hospital. Aero-medical evacuation teams (each consisting of two physicians, three trained nurses and a technician), have been trained at Fairfield Hospital to bring such patients from any part of Australia to Melbourne.

The 1970s seemed to mark the end of major epidemics, with only specific outbreaks of cholera, Murray Valley encephalitis, and typhoid. Over the years Fairfield accepted a more diverse range of patients, and by 1979 the number of principal infectious diseases listed in the annual report had trebled since 1955. This diversity of presenting disease was certainly in evidence in 1978. During 1979, 32 patients with Q fever (caused by a rickettsia that affects many domesticated animals including sheep and goats) were treated. The disease affected meat workers from a number of city and country abattoirs and appeared to be related to the slaughtering of feral goats from Northern parts of Australia; 97 patients who had sera sent to the laboratory were diagnosed with it.

Q fever was by no means the only unusual disease. Diseases originating overseas were making up an increasingly large percentage of hospital admissions. A detailed commentary on 'Imported Diseases' in the 1979 report highlighted the diversity of diseases and their sites of origin in patients admitted to the hospital:

> Forty eight cases of malaria were treated in the twelve month period . . . Twelve adult patients were treated for dengue fever, all of whom had recently returned from overseas . . . There were five cases of leprosy, two were lepromatous, one tuberculoid and two indeterminate. With the exception of one patient, the remainder had acquired their infections outside Australia (Vietnam 2, Hong Kong 1, India 1) . . . All six cases of typhoid fever and seven cases of paratyphoid fever were acquired outside Australia. The sources of the infection in the typhoid fever patients (aged 2–31 years) were India (2), Indonesia (1), Malaysia (1), Malta (1) and South-East Asia (1). Six patients (aged 3–34 years) with paratyphoid A all acquired their disease in South-east Asia (India 3, Philippines 1, Indonesia 1) and one child aged four years acquired paratyphoid B in Turkey . . . A diagnosis of Legionnaires' Disease pneumonia was confirmed in a man aged 56 years . . . He had recently returned from . . . the United States, where he had been warned that he may develop this disease because Legionella pneumonia organisms had been detected in the cooling tower of the hostel at which he had been staying . . . Infection with a group A arbovirus was confirmed in two patients who returned from Fiji in 1979. Both presented with polyarthritis and

rash. Many patients in Fiji presented with similar symptoms in 1979, and preliminary studies showed that the disease was caused by a group A arbovirus
which is closely allied to the Ross River virus (W.H.O. Wkly. Epidem. Rec.,
June 15, 1979). This infection is endemic in Australia where it causes poly-
arthritis, particularly in the North of Victoria.

Other 'miscellaneous infections' included 'milker's nodes', granuloma
inguinale, lymphogranuloma venereum, tetanus, previously uncommon
forms of tuberculosis and lepromatous leprosy. Borderline lepromatous leprosy was confirmed in a 52-year-old man living in north-eastern Victoria.
This man had not been outside Australia, nor had he been in northern

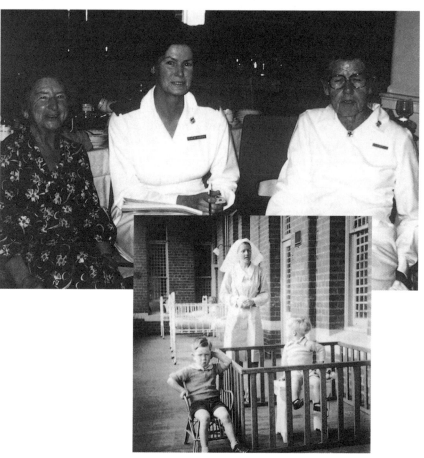

*At the annual reunion of the Past Nurses Association in 1979 are (left to right) Ida Pump,
a fever nurse in the 1940s; Gwen McPherson, Charge Sister and active member of the
Fairfield History Collection Committee, and Edna Yarwood. A younger Sister Yarwood
(below) is on duty in Ward 6 in 1944.*

Dengue fever is an acute infectious viral disease mainly found in Asia and Africa. It is also called 'breakbone', or 'dandy fever'. Several forms of the disease are known: 'classic' dengue, mild dengue and dengue haemorrhagic fever (DHF). Symptoms of classic dengue include fever, severe headache, weakness, skin rashes and severe joint pain (hence the name 'breakbone fever'). Classic dengue is not fatal. The patient is generally very ill for seven days, followed by weakness for many weeks. DHF causes fever, cough, headache, vomiting and abdominal pain. Circulatory collapse and internal haemorrhaging may occur and lead to death. DHF may lead to dengue shock syndrome. DHF is also known as Philippine haemorrhagic fever, Southeast Asian haemorrhagic fever and Thai haemorrhagic fever. Benjamin Rush in America first accurately described dengue fever in 1780, and the cause was demonstrated by P. Ashburn and C. Craig in the Philippines in 1907. The main vector of dengue is the yellow fever mosquito *Aedes aegypti*.

Australia prior to developing the rash. This could be the first documented transmission of leprosy in Victoria. Fungal panophthalmitis occurred in two patients who were drug abusers. They had been using lemon juice to mix up heroin for intravenous injection; two weeks prior to the onset of their symptoms, they had used juice from a mouldy lemon for this purpose. They also had subcutaneous nodules over the face and scalp, presumably of fungal aetiology. A 6-year-old boy who presented with fever, a rash and a healing tick bite on the neck was diagnosed with scrub typhus. He had recently returned from Queensland.

We can close this discussion of the 1970s on a couple of high notes. During 1979 Sister M. Robinson was granted a highly prestigious Churchill Fellowship to study high security infectious diseases in America and Europe. She undertook concentrated studies at the Centres for Disease Control in Atlanta, Georgia, and then visited Coppett's Wood Hospital in London and a number of other specialised infectious disease centres in Britain. She returned to Fairfield in late June, having 'gathered a wealth of nursing information which will guide the nursing department in fulfilling its future responsibilities, both in our present wards and in the new quarantine facility'. Another positive note was the seventy-fifth anniversary of the opening of the hospital

Typhus, an insect-borne, acute—often fatal—infectious disease, was often confused with typhoid. There are several types of typhus, and different forms are transmitted by lice, fleas, (Brill's disease), mites (Tsuganamushi and scrub typhus) and ticks (Rocky Mountain spotted fever, Marseilles fever and South African tick-bite fever). It is caused by species of rickettsia and symptoms include fever, headache and a distinctive rash. In the Middle Ages it was one of many 'pestilences', and it can be recognised in the writings of Spanish doctors of the fifteenth century as '*el tabardillo*'. Louse-borne typhus is associated with overcrowding, and in colonial times was known as 'ship fever' and 'gaol fever'. Typhus was rampant on ships of the Second and Third Fleets arriving in Sydney. In 1852 the government ship *Ticonderoga* arrived in Melbourne; 96 people are recorded as having dying from typhus *en route*, and 80 more died in the quarantine station. Despite the quarantine station, typhus was transmitted to the resident population. Passengers on the *Wanata*, which also arrived in Melbourne in 1852, spread typhus while travelling to the goldfields. Typhus can now be treated by antibiotics. Using insecticides and eliminating overcrowded conditions have also been effective in reducing the incidence of this unpleasant disease.

on 1 October 1904. This auspicious anniversary was celebrated on 10 October. A display of historical material was held in the nurses' recreational hall, and guests and staff were entertained in marquees set up on adjacent lawns. Despite poor weather, the celebration was a great success.

The administrative changes heralded by the appointment of Dr Bennett as Chief Executive Officer gathered momentum towards the end of the decade and continued into 1980. As previously mentioned, these changes led the hospital into a period of great unrest and tension. The Board described the process thus in the 1980 annual report:

> The process of restructuring the administration of the Hospital, which began late in 1978, continued during the last year . . . Suitable appointments were made to the two new positions of Medical Record Administrator and Personnel Officer. Dr Peter Cavanagh was appointed as the administrative head of the laboratory complex and was given the title of Director of Laboratory Services . . . A number of formal committees were established to provide better communication between staff members and the administration. These included a Senior Medical

Staff Committee and Drug, Equipment, Library, Paramedical, Medical Record and Fire and Safety Committees. In addition, the Board subcommittee, the Senior Medical Staff Appointments Committee, was re-established ... Unfortunately in 1980 there was an industrial dispute involving some of the senior medical staff. In order to preserve harmony within the Hospital, the Board of Management resolved to rescind certain decisions it made relating to two of the medical staff. It is hoped that future discussions between the Board and the Medical Staff will lead to more cordial relationships within the Hospital.

The industrial dispute so briefly touched upon in this report was in fact of such intensity and passion that it rocked the hospital to its foundations. Senior medical staff—some of whom had worked in the hospital for many decades—resigned. The basic facts of the dispute are straightforward, but it is difficult to describe the interplay of personal conflicts, professional ambitions, secrecy and suspicion which underpinned the intense passions it generated.

When it first became public knowledge in April 1980, the dispute had already been simmering for some time, Nine of the hospital's senior medical officers submitted their resignations and fourteen members of the Virology Department staff threatened to resign because they believed that Dr Ian Gust, the head of Fairfield's Virology Laboratory and an internationally renowned

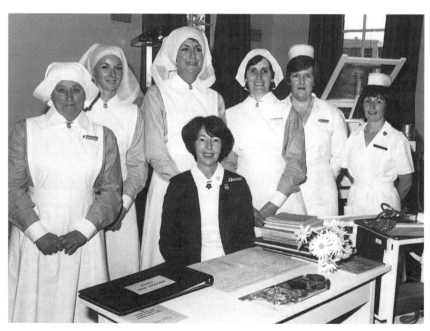

Sister Margaret Leahy (seated) with six nurses in period uniform (1900s to 1960s) at the hospital's seventy-fifth anniversary celebrations in 1979.

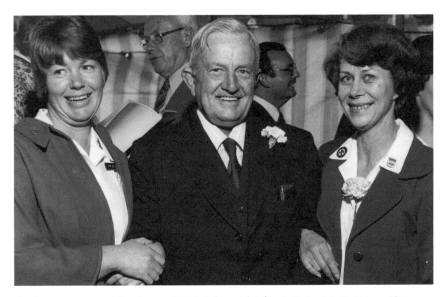

At the anniversary celebrations in 1979 (left to right, front): Sister Marie Brown; Victor Frank, pharmacist; Sister Muriel Dowzef; (back) Bill Marsden, Hospital Secretary; Ron Bever, Catering Officer.

authority in his area, had been treated unjustly by the Board of Management and by the Chief Executive Officer, Dr Noel Bennett. The crux of the problem appears to have been that Dr Gust, a man of considerable drive, charisma, charm and eloquence, and a substantial proportion of his colleagues felt that he was not being allowed to run his laboratory (the high quality of its work was never in question) with the same level of independence that existed prior to Dr Bennett's promotion. The new CEO had worked in the hospital for many years and had been on good terms with his medical colleagues prior to his promotion. He and Dr Gust, while never close friends, had enjoyed an amicable relationship and had even played squash together. Some staff members thought that the problem had its origins in Dr Bennett's apparent belief that his new role meant that he needed to distance himself from his colleagues, or at least to modify existing relationships. The problems between Dr Bennett and Dr Gust were seen by some staff as being largely fuelled by the CEO's desire to stamp his authority on the hospital and to make a clear, public statement that there was no place for independent or even semi-autonomous power bases or leadership roles. There is always the possibility that when a 'new broom sweeps clean' it will try to sweep away that which does not require sweeping and is capable of resisting the attempt. It would be easy to demonise individuals in the dispute and this certainly happened at the time. With the benefit of hindsight one can recognise that the powerful new CEO position created the potential for conflict at a time when management was becoming increasingly pro-active and assertive. (Some might say meddling and aggressive). Put simply, the scenario could be stated thus—if Bennett was going to be undisputed cock of the walk he would have to clip the wings of Dr Gust.

After discussions, the resignations were withdrawn on 28 May. Discussions within the hospital led to establishment of *ad hoc* committees to make recommendations concerning the structure, role and function of the medical staff and the function, structure, role and funding of the laboratories. Each committee comprised representatives of the Board and the medical staff. However, the situation within the hospital remained stormy, and between 26 September and 24 October there were seven resignations. Such disputes within an institution can take on a life of their own, fuelled by rumour and innuendo.

Recognising that the situation was out of hand, the Board—which should perhaps have intervened much earlier—decided that an external circuit breaker was needed. At its request the state government appointed the former ombudsman, Sir John Dillon, to advise the Health Commission on the reasons for the dispute and to propose a course of action for its resolution. Dillon studied many written and verbal submissions from members of staff, Board members, interested individuals and organisations outside the hospital. On 11 December 1980 Dillon's Report was released to the public. Although in essence the report found that there had been faults on both sides, it did state that Dr Bennett was mainly responsible for the deterioration of relationships with the senior staff, noting that he had shown a lack of sensitivity and tact, and that it was the first duty of an administrator to maintain high staff morale. Although to some extent critical of Dr Bennett, Dillon stressed that he was 'a dedicated, hard-working and competent chief executive', and it would be a 'monstrous injustice' if he were to be 'transferred, demoted or dismissed'. Some people at the time regarded the report as rather lenient to the Board. The feeling was that the Board should have been held responsible for the situation that had arisen, as it should have intervened much more effectively before the dispute became acrimonious. Dillon made no less than 114 recommendations designed to resolve the problem, but these did not lead to the withdrawal of resignations.

Dillon had tried hard to bring about a reconciliation between Dr Bennett and the medical staff, even to the extent of organising a meeting—

held only a week before his report was tabled in Parliament. The meeting was not a success, as the *Age* report indicates:

> Sir John sought to bring about . . . a reconciliation between the medical staff and Dr Bennett when he interviewed Dr Bennett on 3 December. But his report shows that Dr Bennett terminated the interview prematurely.
>
> Sir John's report said: 'It had been my intention to put to him his earlier acknowledgement that he would be a "very, very stupid man" if he did not learn from this episode and to consider the possibility of a reconciliation with Dr Gust and other members of the medical staff.'
>
> These doctors were waiting in a nearby room in the State Health Commission offices to shake hands with Dr Bennett but the reconciliation never happened.[5]

Professors S. Faine and R. Pepperell resigned from the Board of Management on 12 January 1981. This was followed by further negotiations with Dr Bennett and the staff members whose resignations had still not been withdrawn, as a result of which Dr Bennett offered to resign as Medical Director and to continue as CEO. The Board accepted this offer but, as Dr Bennett would remain 'in charge' of the hospital, this redesignation did not convince any doctors to withdraw their resignations. Recognising that another impasse had been reached, the Health Commission proposed that Dr Ian Brand be appointed Director of Reconstruction (a role not unlike the Minister of Reconstruction appointed after World War II). Dr Brand was to advise the Board and report on all aspects of the structure and function of the hospital—giving special consideration to those related to the ongoing dispute.

On 17 February Dr Brand was appointed Administrator by the Governor-in Council and assumed all powers of the Board of Management, which was temporarily dissolved. Two days later, Dr Bennett resigned as Chief Executive Officer and Medical Director in order to take up appointment as the hospital's Director of Quarantine Services and Adviser in Infectious Diseases to the Health Commission of Victoria. On 6 May Mr Graeme Houghton was appointed Executive Director—a new position replacing the Chief Executive Officer—and on 13 May Dr Alvis Kucers was appointed Director of Medical Services. At the time it appeared that the main lesson to be learnt from the whole sorry story was that the concentration of medical and administrative powers in the same hands was a recipe for disaster; certainly it had led to some of the hospital's darkest years.

The 1981 annual report presented a very positive commentary—signed by Dr Ian Brand, Administrator, and Graeme Houghton, Executive Director —on the end of the dispute:

> The dispute has been long in duration and has had a deeply divisive effect upon the staff and it is scarcely credible that a resolution could have been achieved

which would have satisfied all parties. Nevertheless, staff morale is high and the Administrator is gratified by the support which he has received and by the support for new administrative processes and appointments which have been implemented. It is the Administrator's view that the hospital is now united and that any residual problems which confront it are quite eclipsed by problems which are external in origin and shared by other public hospitals.

In an attempt to democratise the hospital and, hopefully, avert any further disputes, it was decided to create the position of Chief of Staff.

In the past, the hospital's service has been enhanced by the presence on the staff of Medical Superintendents who have been intensively involved in clinical activities and who have served as a focus for enquires and as spokesmen for the hospital. Following the appointment, for the first time, of a full-time administrative head of the medical Division, it was decided to create the additional position of Chief of Staff. Initially this position will be filled by an elected member of the Medical Staff.

The administrative and medical structure that arose phoenix-like from the ashes of the fiery staff dispute was rather unwieldy and top-heavy:

Organisation Structure Senior Management as at 30 June 1981

Board of Management (temporarily in abeyance as a
result of the staff dispute)—advised by Finance and
Staff Committee, Joint Consultative Committee and
Senior Medical Appointments Committee
↓
Executive Director
↓
Director of Medical Services/ Director of
Administrative Services/ Director of Nursing/
Director of Quarantine Services and Adviser in
Infectious Diseases to Health Commission of Victoria
↓
Chief of Staff (to be appointed)
↓
[Chief of Medical Services, appointed July 1981]
↓
Finance Manager/ Appeals and Publicity Manager

During the whole course of the staff dispute the hospital continued to function effectively, and patients were in no way inconvenienced. In discussing the trends in infectious diseases treated at the hospital during 1980/81, the annual report notes that the period had been 'notable for an absence of large outbreaks of respiratory disease or gastro-enteritis'. There were, however, 9 cases of leptospirosis (Weil's disease), and some 60 patients suffering from golden staph (methicillin-resistant *Staphylococcus aureus* (MRSA)) infections were transferred from other Melbourne hospitals for treatment and care. Imported infections continued to be treated in fairly large numbers: cholera (1), typhoid fever (2), dengue fever (17) and malaria (94)—a record number for the hospital. The period also saw an important advance in the prevention of infectious disease when a vaccine for hepatitis B was tested in United States with a success rate of 92 per cent. The hospital continued its sponsorship of medical aid to Ambon in Indonesia by providing advice and co-ordination to the Gull Force Veterans' Association and the Australian Development Assistance Bureau.

The release in 1981 of the report of the Jamison Inquiry into the Efficiency and Administration of Hospitals had important ramifications for Australian hospitals, particularly when the federal Health Minister drew on some of its 140 recommendations in proposed changes to health funding announced on 29 April 1981. Under these 'reforms' the federal government changed its method of funding hospitals, to a general revenue grant to the states. Other changes to the Medibank health care scheme meant an end to free treatment for uninsured patients in hospital standard beds. These changes forced Fairfield, for the first time in its history, to issue accounts to patients whether or not they had medical insurance. Although the poor and those suffering from some communicable diseases were exempt from these charges, the reforms marked a new era of financial stringency and a 'user pays' mentality.

Of much greater importance to the future development of Fairfield (although no one could have foreseen this) was recognition of the HIV/AIDS epidemic by the United States Centres for Disease Control. The first recorded death from AIDS in Australia occurred on 5 September 1981, the unfortunate victim being a 72-year-old man who was a patient at Sydney's Royal Prince Alfred hospital. The cause of this man's death was not established until November 1993, when a biopsy was undertaken. Of more immediate concern to the hospital at this time was a serious rubella epidemic, which was followed by overlapping epidemics of bronchiolitis and influenza, both B and A, in 1982.

Given the recent turmoil in the hospital, it is not surprising that the 1981 annual report contained a prominent 'mission statement' (to which detail would be added for the 1982 report):

> Recognising that, because of its unique nature, Fairfield hospital operates at state, national and international levels, the objectives of the hospital are:
> 1. To care for people suffering from infectious diseases and the residual effects of infectious diseases;
> 2. To assist in the identification of infectious diseases and in the prevention of their spread in the community;

3. To carry out and promote research related to the aetiology, diagnosis, treatment and prevention of infectious diseases and to the attainment of the Hospital's other objectives;
4. To serve as a centre for the accumulation, development, teaching and dissemination of skills and information relating to infectious diseases;
5. To regularly review the Hospital's objectives to identify other areas of activity to which the Hospital's resources can be applied to the benefit of the community.

As a clash over the running of the laboratory facilities was a central factor in the recent unrest and turmoil, a working party was established to review the structure, role and funding of the Clinical Pathology and Virology laboratories. The working party not only brought their own expertise to bear on their work but also received submissions both from inside the hospital and from interested parties outside. The laboratories had three main functions: service, teaching and research. As well as providing the diagnostic services for hospital patients, they had a state public health function. Following the recommendations of the working party, the Board adopted a charter for the laboratories.

The roles of the Laboratories include:

- provision of a modern and efficient service for the diagnosis of infections of man, the investigation of outbreaks of disease and the detection of potentially pathogenic agents in the environment;
- surveillance of infections in the community. This function includes studies on both hospital patients and patients attending general practitioners or clinics, and involves the collection and analysis of data obtained from these studies, and the maintenance of a representative serum bank. Information on the patterns of infection in the community is to be provided to State and Commonwealth authorities on a regular basis;
- surveillance of the efficacy of immunisation programs in the community;
- working with public health authorities and people in other relevant institutions to devise and evaluate methods for the prevention, treatment and control of infections; assisting in the teaching of health workers; training technologists, scientists and medical graduates;
- conducting research into infections of man;
- the provision of reference facilities for other laboratories in Australia and the Pacific region;
  - collaboration with WHO and other national and international organisations, to play a leading role in the development of laboratory services and the study of infectious diseases in the region.

The official opening of the National High Security Quarantine Unit at Fairfield took place on 5 November 1982 (Guy Fawkes Day—a somewhat inauspicious day to open a new facility). Designated as Ward 18, the new unit was named the Perrin Norris Building in honour of Dr William Perrin Norris (1866–1940), who had played an important role in the development of preventative public health when permanent head of the Public Health Department of Victoria from 1902 until 1912. In explaining the background to the new facility, the 1983 annual report stated:

> Between 1967 and 1976, 3 viral haemorrhagic fevers were recognised for the first time—Marburg virus disease (1967), Lassa fever (1968), and Ebola virus disease (1976). These diseases, endemic in Africa, may be highly infectious and can result in a high mortality. With the increase in travel between nations, there is an increasing possibility of these and other diseases, entering Australia.
>
> Australia's existing quarantine facilities, primarily designed for the isolation of smallpox, were unsuitable for these new diseases. The facilities were old and often remote from specialised medical care and not capable of providing high security containment facilities.
>
> So it was that in 1977 the Commonwealth Department of Health recommended that a National High Security Unit be built and that patients suspected of having one of these diseases be transported by air from anywhere in Australia. This unit would take over the role of the existing facilities located around the Australian coastline.
>
> In recognition of Fairfield's experience in the care, diagnosis and treatment of infectious diseases, it was chosen to house the Unit. In July 1979 the construction began … The Commonwealth Government have funded the complete project—a total of $3.08 million for the ward and laboratory

The hospital had reason to be proud that it was chosen to house this specialised and prestigious national unit. Unfortunately the new unit proved to be something of a poisoned chalice owing to chronic and ultimately irresolvable problems in the design of the building. Due to fundamental design problems in its high-tech air conditioning system, the building would have imploded—destroying the ceiling—if the hospital had tried to operate it as a high-security unit. In fact the unit never fully operated in the role it was designed for, although it did handle one case of suspected Lassa fever and proved useful as a training unit.

The first diagnosed case of AIDS in Australia occurred in Sydney in November 1982. In July of that year, haemophilia-associated AIDS was first reported in the United States.

In what might well be seen as the last step in the healing and reconstruction process following the staff dispute on 24 February 1982, a new Board of Management for Fairfield was announced by the state government—Dr Brand had acted as Administrator for thirteen months. Dr Brand was elected chair of the Board, which consisted of nine men and three women. After an inspection in February by the Australian Council on Hospital Standards,

AIDS is an acronym for Acquired Immunodeficiency Syndrome, the most recent and devastating sexually transmitted disease. It is caused by the human immunodeficiency virus (HIV), now known to be a retrovirus, which was first identified in 1983. HIV is transmitted by body fluids—mainly blood and sexual secretions. It is characterised by failure of the immune system. In Australia, transmission occurs primarily through sexual contact between men. There is a low rate of transmission through heterosexual contact, needle-sharing by illicit drug users, and blood transfusions. The first deaths attributed to AIDS occurred in the United States in 1977.

the hospital was granted full accreditation for the three years ended 26 May 1985. Board and staff were described as being 'delighted and gratified' by this development.

The hospital was then drafting yet another ambitious and foresightful master plan for its development. The plan, based on a comprehensive appraisal of the hospital's present and future role, entailed an extensive and expensive upgrading of the facilities. The Health Commission accepted a copy and expressed an interest in its proposals, but at a time of stringent financial policies the plan was never likely to come to fruition. The hospital administration was fully aware that it was unlikely to receiving any sizeable government funding for upgrading—or even maintaining—the standards of the hospital, and began to focus its attention on other potential sources of funding, particularly charitable community support. In pursuit of this strategy, Sheila Saville was appointed to the newly created position of Appeals and Publicity Manager. Because of its specialist nature the hospital had no geographically circumscribed community support, so Saville's task was a particularly challenging one. This strategy was further developed in 1983 when, as a result of an initiative by Tess Slater, Friends of Fairfield was established. This community support group proved itself to be a worthy successor to the Fairfield Hospital Auxiliary.

In what can be seen as a sign of the times, in 1982 the Board established an interdivisional Computer Advisory Committee to advise on all aspects of data-processing systems and a Bio-safety Committee to ensure the safe application of recombinant DNA technology. The hospital also established a program providing post-graduate experience, normally of about four months duration, in infectious diseases for Fijian doctors and nurses. The first participants in this program, which was fully funded by the Fijian government, were Doctors I. Varea and P. Nadiri and Sisters J. Farouk and K. Teusia. One of the hospital's long-term overseas aid and development programs continued in May 1982 when Dr N. Bennett led a Gull Force Association Advisory Medical Team to Ambon, Indonesia. In the same year Natalie Gedye, a polioneuritis patient at the hospital, became one of the few such patients to give birth while on a respirator. Also in 1982, Dr Ian Gust was appointed Honorary Associate Professor to the Department of Microbiology at the University of Melbourne. He also received two prestigious awards, principally in acknowledgement of his work on hepatitis A virus—the Wellcome Australia Medal and the Selwyn Smith Medical Research Prize.

The increasingly effective mass immunisation programs dramatically reduced the incidence of many of the infectious diseases which in earlier years had provided the bulk of Fairfield's admissions; admissions had been dropping substantially and this trend looked likely to continue. The decreasing demands on the hospital's care and treatment resources provided an opportunity to further develop its research and development strengths. It was in fact brutally clear that if the hospital could not successfully diversify its functions and roles, it had little long-term future. In response to this changing role and to its desire to build upon existing resources and strengths, the Board decided to establish a Medical Research Centre, whose stated aims were:

   (i) promoting improvements in patient care and the development of new measures for prevention and control of infections within hospitals and the community;

  (ii) providing opportunities for medical and science graduates seeking training or careers in medical research;

 (iii) attracting and retaining full-time research workers to the hospital;

 (iv) providing a focal point for the study of infections in the Western Pacific Region.

   The Centre's activities will be funded entirely from grants for particular research projects and from other funds which may become available to support research in general. The Centre will be administered by a sub-committee of the Board.

The hospital managed to win funding of $205 000 from the Health Commission to construct a temporary annexe to the clinical pathology laboratory and a central animal house, reflecting the wisdom of pursuing a greatly expanded research role. The critically important role of medical research was highlighted during the year when researchers at the United States National Cancer Institute and at the Pasteur Institute in Paris isolated the HIV virus (known in France as LAV and in the United States as HTLVIII) that causes AIDS. That the hospital was well positioned to develop its existing

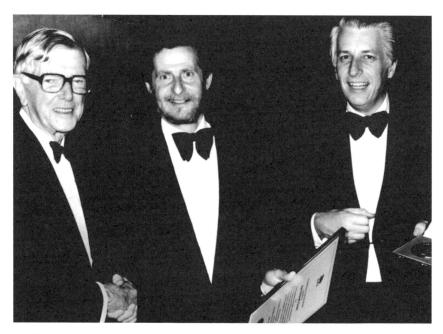

*Professor Ian Gust (centre) after receiving the prestigious Wellcome Medal Australia in
1983, with Sir Macfarlane Burnet (left) and Sir Gustave Nossal.*

research role is suggested by the fact that in December 1983 it hosted a World
Health Organisation Workshop on production of reagents for rapid diagnostic tests of viral infections.

As a result of growing awareness that HIV/AIDS posed a threat of horrific proportions, on 18 November 1984 a federal task force was set up to co-
ordinate the campaign against AIDS. By 1984 Fairfield had already admitted
two confirmed cases of AIDS. The first was a local man aged thirty-two and
the second a US citizen aged twenty-nine who had been diagnosed in the
United States and was admitted to Fairfield when his condition deteriorated
during a holiday in Melbourne. These two unfortunate men were the first of
many hundreds to be admitted to Fairfield over the following years. On the
broader canvas, these young men were part of a worldwide catastrophe of
devastating proportions.

With the government's policy of 'zero growth' in public hospitals entering its seventh year, finance remained an intractable problem for the hospital.
Fairfield complied with the budgetary restraints, but only at the cost of considerable strain and conflicting internal pressures. The most obvious example
of the intense pressures within the public hospital system was the industrial

action undertaken by registered and state-enrolled nurses in 1984. Despite a long history of poor pay and working conditions, nursing staff had traditionally abstained from industrial action. Having finally reached the limits of their endurance and led by progressive and effective union organisers, nursing staff embarked upon a major program of industrial actions, the centrepiece of which was the refusal to undertake any tasks designated as non-nursing duties. This action had a snowball effect within hospitals—including Fairfield—as non-nursing staff took industrial action when ordered to undertake these duties. The nurses' industrial campaign, which had the benefit of widespread support and sympathy in the general community, was resolved after a long struggle on terms generally considered to constitute at least a partial success for the union and its members.

This round of work bans was the precursor of further and increasingly hard-fought industrial campaigns in 1985 and 1986—centred on a log of thirty-three claims presented by the Nurses Federation to the Victorian government on 10 August 1984. For its part the Board of Fairfield went on the public record:

> [We are] gratified that because a constructive approach to the problems was adopted by members of staff and their union representatives, the campaign of industrial action had only a very minor adverse effect on patient care. Notwithstanding the industrial relations conflict referred to, the Board is grateful indeed that the conscientious and often creative initiatives of many members of staff have enabled the hospital to comply with its budget in the year under review.

The Board and senior staff remained deeply concerned that, despite repeated urgent representations to the Health Commission, the hospital still had no agreed formal statement regarding its future role. Management's disquiet about this state of affairs was forcibly impressed upon the Minister for Health when a deputation from the Board lobbied him in January 1984. In May the Board organised a one-day planning seminar attended by members of the Board, senior hospital staff and officers of the Health Commission to explore future development options. Following the seminar, the Board—to no one's great surprise—decided that the hospital should continue to be developed on its present site and to provide 'a comprehensive range of services relating to patient care, teaching and research in infectious diseases and that opportunities should also be sought for the hospital to apply its resources to other public health problems'. This vision of a comprehensive, multi-purpose public health campus at Fairfield was to provide the basic development model for the hospital over the following years.

A *Report on the Capital Requirements of the Publicly Funded Health Services for the Next Ten Years*, prepared by John McClelland, was released in 1984. Although this report did note the state role of the hospital and the need for clearer definition of that role, its concrete proposals were limited to a statement that high priority should be given to redevelopment of the kitchen, clinical pathology, mortuary, outpatients and pharmacy facilities. In response to this rather disappointing report, the hospital argued that a high priority should be given to the urgent need to provide adequate facilities for long-term polio patients and other permanent residents of the hospital. It also noted that the rehabilitation services badly needed rehousing.

Margaret Lafferty, the Director of Nursing, retired at the end of July 1984, having held the position since 1977. The Board paid glowing tribute to her service to the hospital:

> [She was] the latest in a long line of distinguished Directors of Nursing at the hospital. Miss Lafferty has been committed to maintaining and enhancing Fairfield's special contribution to the community and she has worked tirelessly and successfully to ensure that Fairfield's nursing skills and philosophy are preserved and are responsive to the changing demands placed on the hospital. Her term of service as Director of Nursing has been a difficult one and has coincided with financial stringency without precedent in recent decades. To all the challenges that have confronted her she has responded with admirable diligence, competence and dignity and the Board of Management is most grateful for the contribution that she has made to the hospital.

Two interesting changes in different ways influenced the operation of the hospital during 1984. First, in line with plans for regionalisation of the state's hospital facilities, in September the Health Commission appointed eight regional directors to administer health services within the newly defined regional areas. Fairfield came under the North Eastern Metropolitan Region, the Regional Director of which was Dr John Morris. The other change was that in accordance with government policy, the hospital granted a 38-hour working week to all staff except those employed under the determination of the hospitals' remuneration tribunal. This reduction in working hours was warmly welcomed by those staff members who benefited from it. In May 1985 the Australian Council on Hospital Standards inspected the hospital. A few months later the hospital was informed that it had been awarded full accreditation status for a further three years and was congratulated on its general standard of patient care.

Admissions to the hospital in 1984/1985 followed what had become fairly predictable patterns. In winter there was an influx of respiratory infections, bronchiolitis (in babies), croup (in children) and influenza. Spring and early summer brought an increase in the enteroviruses and autumn was, as usual, the hospital's quietest period. Other major reasons for admission included viral hepatitis, gastroenteritis and glandular fever. On a smaller scale, malaria and shingles accounted for a significant number of admissions. A convalescent case of Lassa fever (admitted in January 1985) and a suspected case of the same disease (later found to be malaria) created a flurry of media interest. If this had been the full admission pattern, it would have been very much 'business as usual' at the hospital. That this was not the case was highlighted in the annual report:

> It would seem from the above that the year at Fairfield was not especially remarkable but in reality this was not the case; indeed it is difficult to recall a time when such a view would have been further from the truth. What has made things so extraordinary has been of course, AIDS, a condition which seems destined to dominate the practice of medicine at the hospital for many years to come.

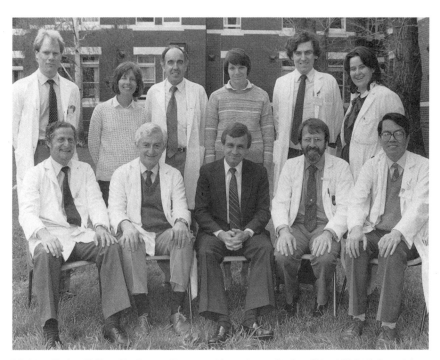

Visiting Forbes Fellow, Dr James Curran, with senior medical staff in 1985: (left to right, seated) Professor Ian Gust, Dr Ron Lucas, Dr Curran, Dr Bryan Speed, Dr Allen Yung, (standing) Dr Richard Doherty, Dr Suzanne Crowe, Dr Murray Sandland, Dr Beverley Biggs, Dr Alan Street, Dr Anna Mijch.

By mid-1984 the hospital was well represented on both the Victorian AIDS Committee and the National AIDS Task Force, and it had cared for two cases of AIDS. In August, serum samples were sent to the Centres for Disease Control, Atlanta, where tests indicated a high rate of infection among homosexual men and persons with haemophilia in Victoria. In September, the development of a Fairfield-based HIV antibody test led to the opening of an AIDS outpatient clinic which provided testing and counselling services to anyone concerned about AIDS. Although there were divisions within the gay community about the wide use of antibody testing, with some leaders advising against testing, the clinic was well patronised. By December, the hospital's virus laboratory had been designated as the national HTLV III reference laboratory. To meet these new responsibilities the hospital employed nine new specialist staff and turned the old animal house into a fully equipped research laboratory. In June, Fairfield was invited to become a World Health Organisation (WHO) collaborating centre for AIDS—one of only three in the world. It was also designated by the WHO as the Biosafety Collaborating Centre for the Western Pacific Region. The ability of Fairfield to draw on its hard-won experience with infectious diseases and its specialised resources was shown by the quality and speed of its response to the AIDS emergency:

> In February and March, the virus laboratory designed and coordinated an evaluation of five commercial kits for the detection of HTLV III antibody. The evaluation which involved five centres including Fairfield, each of whom were provided with 1,000 serum samples and performed 10,000 tests, resulted in the introduction of HTLV III antibody testing in all Australian blood banks and put Australia ahead of the rest of the world in this area, a remarkable achievement.

A remarkable achievement indeed.

The huge level of public interest incorporated significant amounts of alarm, terror and panic, causing misinformation and the spread of rumours. In order to calm these fears, members of Fairfield medical staff gave over a hundred talks on AIDS. The range of groups who sought a speaker from the hospital at this time included ambulance drivers, firemen, policemen, grave diggers, mothers' clubs, Rotarians, lesbian organisations, health-care workers, pharmacists, brothel proprietors and judges.

Even more important than the hospital's research and educational contribution to the onset of the AIDS 'plague' was the provision of care for a further 12 patients with AIDS during 1984/1985. The annual report noted that 'We expect this number to treble or quadruple in the coming year'. This proved a shrewd projection, as the figures rose to 47 AIDS-related admissions in 1985/1986. The horrendous effects of AIDS were reflected not only in the severity of the symptoms but also in an appallingly high mortality rate. By

30 June 1985, 14 AIDS patients had been treated at the hospital—6 had already died, and little hope was held for the survival of the others.

This was indeed a difficult period for the hospital. Struggling with a significant budget shortfall, it was also under pressure as a result of continuing industrial action by the nursing staff over non-nursing duties. In addition, a process to ensure more direct accountability and scrutiny—based on key performance indicators—was put in place by the new regional management.

In an effort to address some of these problems, the hospital introduced a scheme which gave a limited right of private practice to Fairfield's specialist physicians and laboratories. It was hoped that through the creation of a private practice fund, the hospital could afford to purchase some badly needed medical equipment. In relation to a long-term solution, it continued to

> direct its planning energies to the establishment of an organisation similar to the Centres for Disease Control in Atlanta, Georgia, U.S.A. This role model has much to commend it and it is hoped that the health care authorities will recognise the advantages to be gained from such an organisation based at Fairfield.

The Fatal Decade
1986–1996

The past year has seen a firm commitment to continue Fairfield Hospital on its existing site.

Fairfield Hospital Annual Report, 1986, p. 5.

Infectious-disease experts have rounded on the Kennett Government's decision to close the world-renowned Fairfield Hospital.

Age, 11 January 1996.

T HIS IS INDEED the final chapter in the history of Fairfield Hospital. The events detailed, analysed and at times celebrated in the following pages can be seen as a downward spiral towards the closure of the hospital—or perhaps, to use a medical analogy, as a description of the physical decline, debilitating symptoms and terminal illness of a once strong and proud institution. There is unavoidable sadness in the 'death' of a hospital that had served Victoria with great distinction for so many years and, despite the frisson of fear and horror inextricably linked with a 'fever hospital', had won a place in the hearts of the Victorian public. But I will not present a negative 'decline and fall' perspective, but rather attempt to explain the process—medical, economic and political—which resulted in closure. Fairfield Hospital was to a large extent a victim of circumstances; although internal divisions and tensions did play a part in its demise, the factors which led to its dissolution were largely outside its control. My emphasis is on the contribution that Fairfield continued to make to the community and to individual patients right up until its final day, and the courageous and creative struggle mounted by staff, patients and trade unionists to 'Save the Hospital'. We will all respond to the Fairfield story in our own way, depending on our individual political, economic or medical perspectives, but few can doubt the value of the Fairfield story in our understanding of contemporary political and economic developments. It is a story of our times.

A number of developments in 1986—in particular the *Hospital (Powers) Act* 1986 which gave the hospital wider powers to enable it to carry out its objectives—led to a positive statement in the annual report: 'The past year has seen a firm commitment to continue Fairfield Hospital on its existing site. The consequence has been a great lift in morale, a steady improvement in the existing physical facilities and the commencement of major capital projects.' Another development that helped alleviate concerns about the hospital's future was the success of the Fairfield research centre. A formal announcement of the formation of the Macfarlane Burnet Centre for Medical Research (MBCMR) was made by Commonwealth Minister for Health, Dr Neal Blewett, on 22 April 1986. The renaming of the centre was intended to serve as a living memorial to the work of Macfarlane Burnet. Professor Ian Gust was the founding Scientific Director and Dr Richard Doherty the Deputy Director of MBCMR Ltd. The centre operated under its own thirteen-member committee of management, appointed by the Fairfield Board. The objectives of the centre were:

1. To promote improvements in patient care with the development of new measures of prevention and control of infections in hospital and the community
2. To provide opportunities for medical and science graduates seeking training in careers in medical research.
3. To attract and retain full-time research workers to the Hospital.
4. To provide focal point for the study of infections in the Western Pacific Region.

The Centre will co-ordinate research conducted in the Virology Laboratory and will launch a public appeal for funds early in 1987.

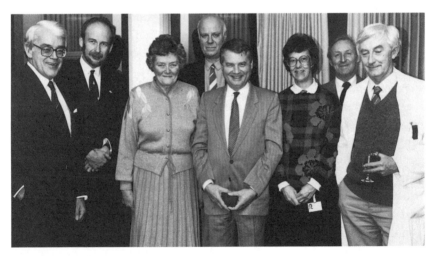

A group of distinguished professors visits the hospital in 1986: (left to right) Geoffrey Connard, Deputy Chairman of the Board; Professor N. Gilmore, Chairman of the Canadian AIDS Taskforce; Marjorie Taylor, Chair of the Board; Dr Alvis Kucers, Director of Medical Services; Professor L. Montagnier of the Pasteur Institute, Paris; Val Seeger, Director of Nursing; Bill Phillips, Executive Director; Dr Ron Lucas, Chief of Medicine.

There was a public launch of the MBCMR Appeal by Prime Minister R. J. Hawke on 30 September 1987. Other pleasing developments during 1986 included the official opening of the New Renal Dialysis Unit on July 30 by Dr John Morris, the North-East Regional Director of Health, and the official openings of the Virology Basement and the Patient Viewing and Re-habilitation Area. On a different, but equally uplifting, note, Giovana Beri, a Fairfield patient, and Nurse Margaret Mitchell were blessed by Pope John Paul II at a celebratory mass held at Flemington Racecourse.

The industrial campaign mounted by the Royal Australian Nursing Federation (and supportive actions by the Hospital Employees Federation) had been simmering for some years; it culminated in a 50-day strike action (31 October – 20 December) late in 1986. Displaying a militancy and solidarity previously almost unthinkable from the ranks of 'professional' nurses, the strike resulted in considerable advances in nursing conditions (a new Registered Nurses Award was handed down on 23 January 1987). It also marked a general recognition that nurses would no longer defer their industrial demands on the grounds of some elevated and disempowering code of professional ethics (read emotional blackmail) or of self-interested assertions

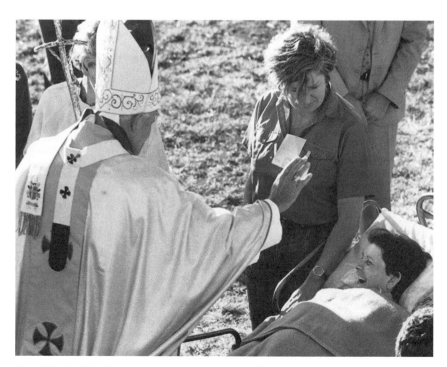

Pope John Paul II blesses patient Giovanna Beri and Nurse Margaret Mitchell at Flemington Racecourse in 1987.

from government and hospital management that improvements in their conditions of employment were not feasible. Commenting on the impact of the strike on the hospital and on the nursing profession, Val Seeger, the Director of Nursing, noted that:

> It was a time of inordinate professional and personal conflict as 'professionalism' was concurrently expressed in habitual nursing or picket line activities. However, it was also the catalyst for nurses to critically re-examine beliefs and values, and for many it heralded a strengthening of commitment and considerable professional growth. During the strike period almost fifty per cent of our registered nurses and a small number of enrolled nurses were absent. The fact that it was possible to resume normal working activities with minimal conflict is indicative of the nurses' determination to restore collegiate relationships and teamwork. This determination has also been reflected in the achievements of the past 6 months.[1]

An outbreak of hand, foot and mouth disease (caused by Coxsackie virus A16) in Melbourne from March to November 1986 caused considerable disquiet. Seventy-four cases were confirmed by the hospital's virus laboratory. This brief episode was relatively insignificant in comparison to the ever-more ominous AIDS epidemic, which continued to challenge the hospital's expertise and resources. One of the hospital's major contributions to the fight against AIDS was the dramatic expansion of its virus laboratory. The number of staff employed at the laboratory more than doubled and extra space was provided through renting a portable laboratory, renovating the old animal house and adding a new basement floor to the existing laboratory building.

Fairfield was, of course, heavily involved in treating people suffering from AIDS and providing an educational resource The extent and complexity of the hospital's response to the AIDS crisis can be seen in a brief contemporary description of its research activities and responsibilities:

> The research, epidemiological and diagnostic aspects of this work have been organised into separate sections—the Special Unit for AIDS Virology, the National Reference Laboratory and the State Reference Laboratory. The Special Unit for AIDS Virology is supported by the Commonwealth Department of Health and is the co-ordinating centre for research teams situated in Melbourne, Sydney, Adelaide and Brisbane. Its budget is $600,000 annually. The main thrust of the team at Fairfield hospital is in the area of research into antiviral agents. The Commonwealth Department of Health is also funding the National Reference Laboratory; based at Fairfield hospital its brief is to compile epidemiological data, evaluate diagnostic tests and reagents, train personnel and advise on difficult technical problems referred by state laboratories. The third of the AIDS laboratories sited at this hospital is the State Reference Laboratory, which is funded by the Health Department of Victoria and its function is the diagnosis of patients within Victoria and the correlation of statistics for the state.[2]

In 1987 Fairfield became one of five partners in the Australian Medical Research and Development consortium (AMRAD). This corporation was established by the state Labor government to help ensure that the benefits of innovative local research remained within Australia. Dr John Stocker was appointed as Managing Director of the corporation on 30 September 1987.

Disease patterns during 1986/87 remained unexceptional: confirmed cases of influenza were the lowest since 1957, and other diseases were described by phrases such as 'relatively mild', 'a small number' and 'moderate numbers'. AIDS, however, continued to take a terrible toll and made heavy claims on the hospital's resources, as the 1987 annual report noted: 'AIDS again dominated the practice of medicine at Fairfield hospital in many ways. Whilst in June 1986, the hospital had cared for 38 category A AIDS patients, by June 30 1987, the total number of such patients was 85, an increase of 124 per cent during the last 12 months.' The hospital's prominent role in the fight against AIDS was acknowledged with the appointment of Ian Gust as deputy chair of the National AIDS Task Force, and the hosting by the World Health Organisation, Western Pacific Region, of an HIV Laboratory Workshop (attended by nineteen delegates from throughout the region) at Fairfield on 24 July 1987. In an incisive summary exploring many aspects of the AIDS epidemic, Dr Ron Lucas, Chief of Medicine, senior physician and a specialist in AIDS at the hospital, stated in the annual report:

> All cases during the last 12 months occurred in homosexual or bisexual men as was the case last year. In addition to the cases of AIDS there are over 1,000 gay men known to have positive HIV antibody tests in Victoria and unless an effective treatment is developed, it is certain that the number of new cases among them will continue to increase for at least the next two years.
>
> Except for persons with haemophilia, the prevalence of infection remains low among other risk groups. For instance positive HIV antibody tests have been found in only 20 out of the approximately 4,000 intravenous drug users tested. In the United States and other Western countries infection in this group has not only been of importance in its own right but also because it has been a major source for heterosexual transmission and in turn, through the infection of child bearing women, of transmission to babies and infants. Fewer than twenty females in Victoria are known to have positive antibody tests and so long as this situation continues it can be predicted that paediatric infection will not increase significantly beyond the small number of children already infected as a result of transfusion of blood or blood products prior to the introduction of donor testing in 1985. Even if infection were to spread rapidly among groups other than gay men, because of the long incubation period, it would be some years before cases of AIDS among them added greatly to the total.
>
> The increased case load during the year has lead [*sic*] to an increased demand for beds. This has been met to a large extent by earlier discharge from the ward than used to be the case with the completion or continuation of a treatment

course being undertaken in a day centre . . . The day centre concept is liked by the patients who prefer to spend as much time as possible at home and there is still plenty of scope for its further development resulting in shorter inpatient stays and considerable cost-savings.

It was becoming increasingly clear that the AIDS epidemic was so virulent and pervasive, so resistant to existing treatment interventions, that the prospects of any diminution of its terrible toll, let alone a 'cure' or effective preventive response, were extremely poor. In the medium and perhaps even the long term, AIDS was here to stay; and in all likelihood the epidemic would get worse, perhaps much worse, before it got better.

An important initiative during 1987 was the formation in March of the Fairfield Hospital Historical Collection Committee. Its objective was to set up a museum to illustrate the unique history of the hospital through a display of the many interesting items amassed since its opening in 1904. There were nine members on the original committee, with Dr Bryan Speed (chair), Barbara Wright (secretary) and M. Bercloux (honorary curator) being the principal office-bearers. The committee found a home for the large collection in the hospital's southern annexe, and set about the formidable task of sorting and recording it. The committee was fortunate to have the unstinting and knowledgeable assistance of Gwen MacPherson and Vera Westley, both of whom were retired Fairfield nursing sisters, and the advice and support of the Executive Director, Bill Phillips. In the following years the Historical Collection developed into one of the most extensive and well-organised of its kind in the world.

The year 1988 was Phillips' last full year of service as Executive Director of the hospital—he resigned in 1988 and was replaced by Chris Richards. It was a fruitful year for the hospital. The newly refurbished kitchen was opened by the Minister for Health, Caroline Hogg, on 13 January; the refurbished Intensive Care Unit and Radiology Department was opened by Dr Neal Blewett on 17 June 1988; and the new Pathology Building (which had been functioning since May) was officially opened by the Premier of Victoria, John Cain, on 14 July. The MBCMR Appeal (launched in September 1987) reach its target of $2.3 million by Easter. In October the hospital was again—after a rigorous survey—awarded full three-year accreditation status by the Australian Council on Hospital Standards. This was the third time in succession that the hospital had won this prestigious status.

The continuing AIDS crisis continued to loom as a dark cloud over the hospital—and indeed the whole community. Lucas reported:

During the twelve months to June 30, 1988, 83 newly diagnosed cases of AIDS were treated at the hospital, almost double the number that had occurred in the previous twelve months. All but three of the patients were homosexual or bi-sexual men. Two of those with other risk factors were women who had sexual contact with bisexual men and the third was a male ex-intravenous drug user whose infection had been acquired overseas.

A worthwhile joint initiative between Fairfield and the Victorian AIDS Council during the year was the construction of a garden retreat in the grounds. This beautifully landscaped retreat provided a much-needed place of sanctuary and tranquillity for AIDS patients and was also used as a meeting place for patients and their visitors.

Disease patterns during 1988/89 reflected a somewhat different pattern from the previous few years: there was a major outbreak of viral meningitis during the summer and an epidemic of Ross River fever. The latter began in East Gippsland in early November 1988 and had spread to most parts of Victoria by the end of the year; it remained a problem, although a steadily diminishing one, into the middle of 1989. AIDS, however, continued to dom-inate the work of the hospital. In 1988/89, 99 people with newly diagnosed cases of full-blown AIDS were admitted. While this was by no means a reduc-tion, indeed it was 16 more than the previous year, the fact that the increase was 'only' 19 per cent reflected a considerable improvement over the last few years when admissions had doubled or worse each year. As in previous years, nearly all the new patients were homosexual or bisexual men; only two were women. Surprisingly, there were no new cases among people whose only known risk factor was intravenous drug use.

For a variety of reasons the slowing down of the rate of increase in AIDS admissions did not remove very much pressure, as the annual report in 1989 noted:

> In spite of the decline in the rate at which new cases were diagnosed the demands on staff and the Hospital's resources continue to increase. Because of improved treatment of opportunistic infections and the use of the antiviral drug zidovudine the survival of AIDS patients is now better than it was, and during the year the increase of 'still alive' patients, on whom workload depends, was greater than the increase of new patients.
>
> As a result the AIDS ward was almost always full and the number of patients who had to be admitted to other wards was sufficiently high that the opening of a second AIDS ward has become a priority

The exponential—and tragic—growth in demand for beds in the AIDS ward forced the hospital not only to begin work on a second AIDS ward but also to plan the renovation of a third for the exclusive use of AIDS patients. Fairfield was justifiably proud of its response to the AIDS epidemic, noting in the 1989 annual report that 'The AIDS unit under the direction of Ron

Lucas, ably supported by Murray Sandland, Anne Mijch, and sessional staff provides a service in the management of AIDS patients acknowledged by outsiders as second to none in the world'. But management and senior medical staff were 'mindful of the danger that Fairfield may be known primarily as an AIDS hospital'. To counteract this tendency to view Fairfield in a restricted and indeed inaccurate light, the hospital went to great lengths to stress its 'role as a centre of excellence' in relation to 'all Infectious Diseases'.

Given this concern that the hospital would be pigeon-holed as a single-disease specialist hospital, one can understand the delight it expressed when the state government announced that it intended to establish the Victorian Infectious Diseases Epidemiology Unit at Fairfield. Among other things, this initiative would enable the hospital to develop an upgraded computing capacity. It was widely seen as being a pat on the back for the hospital's excellent work in responding to the AIDS epidemic. From the hospital's point of view, being chosen as the site for the new epidemiology unit was recognition of its continuing role as *the* infectious disease hospital in the state (and indeed in the nation).

The Macfarlane Burnet Centre for Medical Research continued to thrive, becoming incorporated as a separate legal entity on 28 December 1989. The role of this important research centre—which was very much part of the vision of Fairfield developing as a comprehensive public health campus—was succinctly described in its first annual report:

> The Centre, which is committed to research into virus diseases which pose significant public health problems, is the largest centre of its kind in Australia.
>
> The Centre works closely with the World Health Organisation and other international agencies, including AIDAB, to assist in the study and control of virus diseases in South East Asia and the Western Pacific and to train scientists from the region. The Centre maintains strong links with the National Institutes for Health, and Centres for Disease Control in the United States, and similar bodies in Europe and the United Kingdom.
>
> *Aims and Objectives of the Centre:*
> The aims of the Centre are to conduct research into virus infections of public health importance, in particular
> • To understand how viruses produce disease and the way in which it is spread.
> • To develop improved methods for the diagnosis, treatment and control of the major virus infection of the Western Pacific Region.
> • To conduct research and train workers in the field on infection and its control, to work with other members of the health profession on the application of the Centre's research thereby resulting in improved patient care.
> • To Provide opportunities for medical and sciences graduates in medical research and maintaining a focal point for the study of infections in the Western Pacific Region. Our immediate objectives are:

- To maintain research units concerned with the pathogenesis, epidemiology, diagnosis and prevention of viral diseases of man.
- To construct a building to provide adequate, facilities for the research units and laboratories for visiting scientists and graduate students.
- To become largely self funding through a combination of external grants, public support and commercially contracted research work.

One of the highlights of 1988/89, was the opening of the new Out-patients Clinic (the old Pathology Building, restored and given a new lease of life) by the Minister for Health, Caroline Hogg, on 9 June 1989. Another notable event, listed in the 1989 annual report in a section entitled 'Highlights of the Year', was the 'Purchase of additional freezer capacity for our mortuary'. On Australia Day 1990, Dr Noel Bennett, Director of Quarantine Services, was named Victorian of the Year and presented with a plaque by Premier John Cain, who commended Dr Bennett for his outstanding contribution to public health in Victoria.

Dr Lucas and his co-workers in the AIDS unit were pleasantly surprised when, contrary to predictions, there was a substantial fall in the number of new cases in 1989/90. Seventy-one cases were diagnosed, compared to 108 and 90 in the two previous years. Past experience and current scientific research on AIDS had led the unit to expect a progressive increase for several more years, probably until 40 to 50 per cent of all infected persons in Victoria had contracted the full-blown disease. As of 31 March 1990, 389 cases of AIDS had been reported to the Victorian Health Department. This figure represented only 17 per cent of the 2310 people known to be infected, according to the Health Department of Victoria AIDS/HIV Surveillance Programme Summary Report, 30 April 1990. Although a variety of factors may have played a part in the drop in diagnosis, medical staff in the AIDS unit believed that the downward trend probably resulted from the introduction of more effective medical management programs. This was exciting, for if this was indeed the case it was possible that AIDS/HIV could become a manageable chronic infection rather than a death sentence.

The encouraging decrease in the number of new cases—from a peak of 108 cases in 1988/89—did not, of course, immediately reduce the pressure on the AIDS unit. The hospital's much-needed second HIV unit (Ward 16) was opened by Health Minister, Caroline Hogg, on 9 March 1990. Although up to half of all inpatients at Fairfield were suffering from AIDS, we must avoid the temptation to see the other aspects of the hospital's work as side issues. The hospital remained committed to providing a comprehensive range of world-quality infectious disease services—treatment, care, research, professional training, public education etc. Under the leadership of Chris Richards, the vision of Fairfield as a centre of excellence for infectious diseases and public health had become even more pronounced. Indeed, there was a persuasive school of thought which saw a multi-faceted public health campus at Fairfield as the only development that could ensure the future of the hospital. The dramatic expansion of the hospital's outpatient and travel services points to the responsiveness of the hospital to changing demands.

The outpatients service had grown from a few follow-up clinics for recently discharged patients to a formal service which catered for both previous inpatients and people who had never before been to the hospital. The number of people seeking pre-travel health advice and various immunisations reflected the increasing number of Australians travelling abroad. In 1983 only about 5–6 per cent of the Australian population travelled overseas in one year; by 1988 almost 1.7 million overseas trips were taken by Australian residents—about 10 per cent of the population. Due to increased demand for pre-travel health service, in 1989 several outpatient clinics were designated as Travel Clinics. After a review of the travel service early in 1990, this was increased to five clinics per week and Dr Tilman Ruff was appointed to the new post of Director of Health Travel. A telephone advice service to the public, staffed by two senior sisters, was trialled for several months in the second half of 1989. The average number of calls was between 45 and 60 per day. However, this service was discontinued after the trial period for lack of sufficient staff. Fairfield staff also ran travel health seminars and produced a number of information pamphlets on aspects of travel health.

The resources invested in the travel service by the hospital can be well understood by looking at just one infectious disease—typhoid fever. Between January 1988 and June 1990, 23 cases of typhoid fever were admitted to Fairfield. Of these patients, only three contracted the infection in Melbourne; the others caught it while travelling overseas. The global village provides many advantages for humankind, but lurking in the background lies the very real danger of rapid transmission of infectious diseases.

The optimism felt about the AIDS epidemic was short-lived, for 107 new cases of Category A AIDS were diagnosed at Fairfield in 1990/91. Significantly, 60 new cases were diagnosed in the second six months of this period, the highest number of new cases treated in any six-month period since the onset of the epidemic. The AIDS unit's analysis of this disappointing upward trend was that it most likely did not represent a new wave in the epidemic, but was linked to a quickening progression to full-blown AIDS as the effectiveness of treatments based on AZT declined.

The resurgence of new AIDS admissions was not the only dark cloud hanging over the hospital as it moved into the 1990s. The internal divisions which so beset the hospital at the start of the 1980s—which had eventually led to the removal of the Board and a radical restructuring of senior management —pale into insignificance when compared to the internal divisions and external threats which were to blight, undermine and finally destroy Fairfield in the 1990s. Fairfield's future had never really been secure at any time since it opened in 1904. At various times—the peak or immediate aftermath of major epidemics—it was less insecure than usual, but it was never really a certain bet to remain functioning from one year to the next. It is probably a fair comment that had it not been for the AIDS epidemic, the hospital might well have closed during the mid-1980s.

The 'golden age' of fever hospitals was the 1920s and 1930s. When epidemics of diphtheria, scarlet fever, measles, whooping cough and meningitis were commonplace, Fairfield often had bed occupancy rates of 500 or more per month. With the dramatic decline of diphtheria, the effectiveness of new wonder drugs such as penicillin, the effectiveness of vaccinations and improved general health and hygiene standards, these levels of bed occupancy had been falling since the 1940s. By 1990 the average rate was only 73 (most of whom were AIDS patients). A total of 160 beds was available, of which only about 100 were 'staffed' functioning beds. Clearly the 1990s shaped to be the most challenging and dangerous years ever faced by the hospital.

Even with a completely united and harmonious staff working in tandem with an effective and supportive Board of Management, Fairfield would have struggled to survive the 1990s; that this was seldom, if ever, the case certainly sealed its fate. The resignation of Dr Ian Gust, Director of the Macfarlane Burnet Centre and the federal government's chief medical adviser on AIDS, on 28 August 1990 was a devastating blow not only to the status and morale of the hospital but also, arguably, to its long-term viability. Dr Gust had served the hospital with the greatest distinction for some twenty-five years and it would be hard to overstate the impact of his departure. It came about, at least in part, as a result of a conflict with hospital management. Gust felt that money raised for the Macfarlane Burnet Centre should be dedicated to the work of the Centre rather than, as he alleged, being seen as general hospital revenue. The dispute provided a focus for existing tensions between the medical staff and hospital management. The extraordinarily high level of popular support for Dr Gust within the hospital was taken up by the media. The *Age* reported that 'staff feelings over his resignation were running so high that when Dr Gust walked to a conference room on Friday for his meeting with the board, scores of staff greeted him outside with three cheers'. The depth of dissatisfaction and division within the hospital at this time led one 'senior medical officer' to tell a reporter: 'The hospital is really in a very dangerous position at the moment. It has a very low bed-occupancy rate (although a large outpatients' service) and demoralised staff . . . It is likely that it will be closed down . . . or amalgamated.' Ominously, 'senior staff' were said to be putting forward the view that 'amalgamation with another hospital in the region might be a way out of the hospital's difficulties'.[3]

In the wake of Dr Gust's resignation, a 'confidential' report by Dr Geoff Dreher, a former executive director of Royal Melbourne Hospital, contained an extremely critical assessment of the management of Fairfield. Management felt that this report was very 'one-sided' and failed to take into account the reasons behind the changes that had been instituted. The closure of fully staffed wards which had few patients but were 'waiting for the epidemic—which didn't occur' were cited by management as examples of ill-informed criticism from medical staff.

Rumours about the closure of the hospital were gaining currency, and causing considerable disquiet within the hospital, by the early part of the year. These fears were compounded in February 1991 when a report on the impact of integrating Heidelberg Repatriation Hospital into the state health system, jointly commissioned by the Victorian Health Department and the federal Department of Veterans Affairs, recommended the closure of Fairfield. Following this report and persistent rumours regarding the closure of the hospital, Peter Grant, president of the Victorian AIDS Council, urged the Minister for Health to make a public announcement about Fairfield's future. Describing Fairfield as 'leading the way in HIV/AIDS treatments and research in Australia', Grant expressed concern about rumours that the hospital was to be closed and stated that '90 per cent of Victorians who were HIV positive were using the services at Fairfield because other hospitals did not offer the same quality of care'. Although the AIDS Council was supportive of the government's policy of providing treatment for infectious diseases in all major public hospitals, it was concerned about unsatisfactory procedures in many public hospitals and believed that no consideration should be given to closing Fairfield until other hospitals came up to Fairfield's standard.[4] The Minister for Health responded to the AIDS Council's request, stating that there were no immediate plans to close Fairfield but that a decision on its future would be made within a year. During the months which followed, as Fairfield faced what we might call its first threat of closure, the support of the Victorian AIDS Council was of critical importance and may indeed have tipped the balance in saving the hospital.

Two major articles on the future of the hospital appeared in the *Age* on 22 May 1991. One contained extremely strong comments from three of Fairfield's senior medical staff—Dr Suzanne Crowe, Dr Anne Mijch and Dr

Ron Lucas. Lucas, who was Chief of Staff of Medicine (and a widely respected authority on AIDS treatment and care), said that the ethos that had made the hospital so successful was under threat: 'There're two camps, medical and management and that means morale is terrible. People are terrified we are about to close up.' Lucas had served Fairfield with great distinction and commitment for over thirty years, pioneering the development of the Renal and AIDS Unit and its hepatitis research. The depth of his unhappiness was evidenced some nine months after this article appeared, when he resigned from the hospital. The second article confirmed Lucas' worst fears: Health Minister Maureen Lyster announced that Fairfield was to be closed. On the face of it, the decision seemed unequivocal. A three-month review was to be set up under Professor Tania Sorrell, head of the HIV unit at Westmead Hospital, New South Wales, and Professor Peter McDonald of Flinders Medical Centre, South Australia, to work out the exact timing and logistics of the closure. Fairfield appeared to have reached the end of the road.

Fairfield was not, however, going to roll over and die quietly like an old dog. Over a hundred staff members attended a hurriedly called emergency meeting on 22 May and vowed to oppose the closure. Within a week, key health unions had met at Trades Hall Council to plan union opposition. Over 500 union members representing some 15 unions, and other supporters of the hospital, attended a meeting at Fairfield on 6 June (appropriately enough, perhaps, the anniversary of D Day) to discuss how best to fight the closure. At the meeting, trade unionists, patients (through consumer organisations such as the AIDS groups and the Ventilator User Network) and community organisations agreed to join forces. This decision led to the formation of the Save Fairfield Committee, which played a crucial role in the campaign to save the hospital.

On 7 June the Health Minister was reported to have moved away from earlier statements that the Sorrell/McDonald review presupposed the closure of Fairfield, stating that the government was not locked into any position on the future of the hospital.[5] In the following months, letters supporting the retention of the hospital appeared in the press with great regularity, and a wide variety of pro-retention submissions were made to the infectious diseases review—including a powerful submission from the hospital's Senior Medical Staff Association and one from the Victorian AIDS Council urging that the role of Fairfield should be expanded to include respite, palliative and hospice care.

A mass rally of over 1000 patients, staff and supporters marched from the city square to Parliament House on 5 September to protest the decision to close Fairfield. The rally culminated in a delegation presenting the Minister

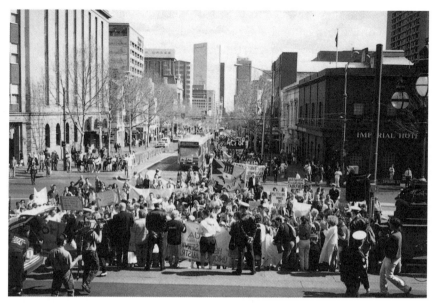

The Save Fairfield Hospital rally on the steps of Parliament House in September 1991.

for Health with a petition, signed by 100 000 people, demanding the retention of Fairfield. Personal testimony was given by Joan Gillespie—one of the
hospital's 'oldest' and most loyal patients. Stricken with polio at the age of
twenty-two, she had once lived at Fairfield for fifteen years and still required
a ventilator for fourteen hours a day. She stated simply that she supported
Fairfield because 'it has kept me alive all these years'.[6] Such accounts helped
to ensure that public opinion was strongly behind the campaign.

The campaign to save Fairfield had no influence on the findings of the
Sorrell/McDonald review. Published early in October, it recommended—to
no one's great surprise given its terms of reference—that all clinical services
at Fairfield be transferred to 'more appropriate sites'. The findings of the
review were disappointing to Fairfield's supporters, but their hopes were raised
when the government announced that a three-month period of public consultation would follow the review's release. At the end of October the Health
Minister announced that the government was considering amalgamating
Fairfield and the Austin Hospital.

The breadth of support was effectively demonstrated at Fairfield on
14 November when a well-publicised meeting of representatives from
throughout the health industry—including the traditionally conservative

Australian Medical Association and the left-leaning Health Services Union—agreed to form a coalition to fight for the retention of Fairfield. Within Fairfield itself, however, there were deep divisions: the Board of Management and the Executive Director supporting components of the Sorrell/McDonald review that some staff felt would destroy the hospital's ability to provide a viable clinical service.

Some 3000 Fairfield supporters marched through Melbourne on 1 December in a protest organised by the AIDS lobby group, Act Up. The protesters confronted the Health Minister as she attempted to present the opening address at an AIDS benefit held to mark World AIDS Day. Lyster informed the protesters that Fairfield's funding had been guaranteed for the next year, that HIV-positive people would be consulted on the redefinition of the hospital's role, and that the government had 'pledged that Fairfield will continue as a research and clinical facility'.[7] Fairfield supporters felt that the tide had turned. This was confirmed when the state government, as a result of the consultative process, stated that Fairfield would continue to provide clinical services; that it supported the establishment of Fairfield Institute for Infectious Diseases, and that infectious diseases treatment services in general hospitals would be enhanced.

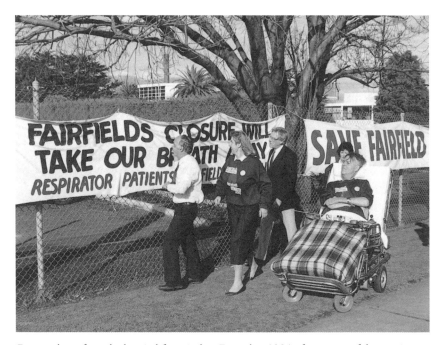

Banners hang from the hospital fence in late December 1991 after a successful campaign. Patients and staff wear windcheaters proclaiming 'Fairfield Hospital: Beyond 2000'.

The Health Department, Fairfield Hospital and the Victorian Trades Hall Council met in January 1992 to discuss implementing the government's decision on the retention of Fairfield. The meeting resolved that Fairfield would be maintained as a viable public hospital; that the total level of resources available to Fairfield Hospital would be guaranteed for infectious diseases services in Victoria; that a Central Steering Committee would be established to oversee the implementation process, and that the impact of any changes affecting staff at the hospital would be implemented through the Statewide Retraining, Redeployment and Redundancy Agreement process.

The Fairfield Hospital Steering Committee comprised representatives from the Hospital Board, the staff, the Save Fairfield Hospital Action Committee, the unions and the Health Department. It presented its final report in July 1992. Its recommendations—which were accepted by the state government—were that Fairfield bed numbers be reduced from 154 to 138; that the 40 HIV/AIDS dedicated beds remain and include 10 beds for palliative care; that a formal link be established between the Austin Hospital and Fairfield; that $2.3 million saved through efficiencies at Fairfield be allocated to the Alfred Hospital, where HIV/AIDS beds would be increased from 9 to 21; that 40 beds at Fairfield be reserved for patients with acute infectious diseases; that 4 beds be reserved as intensive-care beds; that the respiratory ward be enlarged from 15 to 19 beds; that Fairfield's 20-bed convalescent-stroke ward be closed; and that the day-care unit be scaled down from 20 to 15 patients. Dr Bryan Speed, writing on behalf of senior medical staff in the 1992 annual report, reflected the general attitude: 'It was with some trepidation that the Medical Staff entered into the processes of the Steering Committee but ultimately the outcome was as favourable as we could have hoped with the retention of a viable clinical service of 138 beds'. He described the agreement reached with the Health Department as a plan to 'retain, re-structure and revitalise the [hospital's] clinical services'.

The successful battle to 'Save Fairfield' by staff, patients and community supporters had been hard-fought. It was only as a result of an extraordinarily committed and united campaign that the hospital's supporters managed to snatch victory from the jaws of defeat. Given the volatile nature of the health industry, and the political and economic climate, those who recognised the outcome of the campaign as a reprieve, a stage in an ongoing struggle rather than a conclusive victory, were wise.

During all of the drama, the normal life of the hospital continued: patients were treated and cared for, research was undertaken, community education and liaison went on. There were indeed a number of interesting developments—unrelated to the closure threat—during the period. In 1991

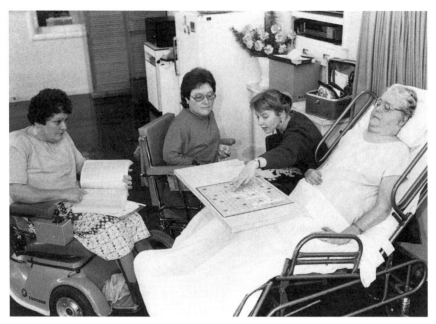

June Middleton (right), a long-term polio patient, was very active in the social life of the hospital and in the campaign to save it.

the National Centre for Health Program Evaluation became a 'tenant' on the hospital campus. Ironically, this was a centre for excellence in the area of health economics. In another positive development in May 1991, the hospital's entero-respiratory laboratory was designated by the World Health Organisation as one of two Western Pacific Region Reference Laboratories for the diagnosis of poliomyelitis. Kerri-Ann Brussen was appointed to carry out the functions of the laboratory. Attracting such tenants and extending the hospital's research responsibilities and facilities formed part of the vision, shared by the Board and Executive Director, Chris Richards, of a multifaceted public health campus providing a focus for all aspects of public health—research, education, consumer groups and professional organisations. This vision did not necessarily encompass a clinical service on campus and this, of course, was one of the principal causes of disharmony and distrust. Some staff were committed to the retention of a major clinical service—what many would have described as a 'real hospital'—while others embraced the vision of a public health campus. The latter scenario contained a good deal of realism, and the arguments that supported it had substance.

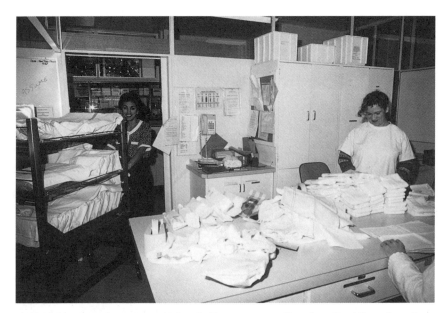

Behind the scenes, charge nurse Helen Goble removes a trolley of sterilised linen from the Central Surgical Services Department.

One visible—and, to many nurses, welcome—change occurred in 1991. An updated uniform policy was introduced in January, 'marking a further significant change in recognition of changing infection control and industrial practices'. Nurses' uniforms are no longer provided, or laundered, by the hospital, and staff now had considerably greater flexibility in their choice of uniform. This change was implemented quickly and without dissent. More important was the publication in August of the hospital's Equal Opportunity Policy, as required by law. It stated that:

> It is the policy of Fairfield Hospital to establish and implement an Equal Employment Opportunity Program. In accordance with the Public Authorities (Equal Employment Opportunity) Act, 1990, EEO for women will be the first priority. The program's aim will be to eliminate, as far as practicable, all discrimination against women in and entering the workforce and to ensure that all employees and applicants for employment are treated fairly and on merit, without regard to their gender.

The resignation in February 1992 of Dr Ronald Lucas, a leading authority on HIV/AIDS and one of Fairfield's most senior and highly respected doctors, got the new year off to a bad start: Dr Lucas' resignation was a protest against aspects of Fairfield's administration. A newspaper report, published the day after his resignation became public, presented a rather inflammatory account of his reasons:

> Dr Lucas quit because he believed administrators driven by budgetary considerations encroached on patient care.
>
> He said too much was spent on management, and not enough on medical services.
>
> 'They made it difficult for me to do my job properly,' he said.
>
> His stand was backed by senior Fairfield staff, who yesterday blamed what they called an incompetent and uncaring management for his resignation.[8]

The departure of a doctor of Dr Lucas' stature would at any time have been a great loss to the hospital; to lose him at this juncture and for the reasons he expressed was a major blow. The support his principled stand received from his fellow staff members demonstrated that no rapprochement had taken place between management and medical staff in the wake of the campaign to save the hospital. This did not bode well for the future.

Another ominous event occurred on 3 October 1992 when at the state elections the conservative coalition won a landslide victory and the Liberal Party's Jeff Kennett replaced Labor's Joan Kirner as Premier. Within a couple of months of winning office, the Kennett government, great believers in so-called market economics and economic rationalism, had introduced such radical and controversial changes to industrial relations legislation that Melbourne witnessed protest rallies the like of which had not been seen since the Vietnam Moratorium demonstrations in the 1970s. Unlike the previous Labor governments under Cain and Kirner, which had been responsive to public opinion and lobbying from interest groups, the new government had a radical right-wing political agenda; it soon showed itself to be both energetic and single-minded in its efforts to introduce changes and to make dramatic cuts to expenditure. As we shall see, the new government was to have a profound effect on the hospital over the next few years.

Fairfield entered into a service agreement with the Macfarlane Burnet Centre in 1992, covering the range of services provided by the hospital to the centre. The centre was also given permission to refurbish the former Wards 15 and 16 as a laboratory. This initiative was seen as strengthening the close medical and scientific links that already existed between the two organisations (although these links, as we have seen, were not always altogether harmonious) and relieved the space pressure in the Virology Department where the research centre was housed.

The AIDS epidemic continued to be by far the most pressing of the hospital's clinical concerns. In 1991/92, 115 new cases of AIDS were diagnosed, there were 313 Victorian notifications of new HIV positive people, and 250 new HIV positive patients attended Fairfield. The cumulative total of AIDS patients treated at Fairfield Hospital by 30 June was 592 (588 men and 10 women) and the cumulative numbers of HIV patients attending Fairfield was 1506 (90 per cent of total cumulative Victorian HIV notifications).

Dr Anne Mijch from the AIDS Unit presented this summary of its work and services in the 1992 annual report:

> Over the past twelve months the service at Fairfield has consolidated into two inpatient ward areas and daily outpatient services, including two evening clinics. A large day-care facility operating five days a week for infusions, transfusions and day surgery also forms part of the HIV service. Ancillary services include counselling, a methadone program for HIV positive patients, a full range of social work services and pastoral care. The HIV service has an active Clinical Research department allowing patients access to the newest agents available for therapies and at the same time scientific review and analysis adds to the pool of knowledge about the management of HIV infection and its opportunistic complications.

A new Continuing Care Unit was opened at the hospital on 7 December 1992. This unit had ten beds and was located on the second floor of the block wards. Care was provided by an interdisciplinary team who collaboratively devised care and management plans for each patient. Both respite care (to support home care-givers) and palliative care (reduction in symptoms and improved quality of life) were provided to people who had reached advanced stages of HIV disease.

Valerie Seeger, the Director of Nursing, resigned in July 1992 'after 30 years of service and an outstanding contribution to many areas of the hospital, including the professional advancement of nurses'. Peg Higginbottom was promoted to the position. Given the interest that Sister Seeger had always taken in the training and professional advancement of nurses, she would have been pleased to see that the year of her retirement also marked the establishment of a Nursing Research Unit on the campus.

Depending on one's point of view, the fact that the 1993 annual report prefaced its medical services report with Giuseppe di Lampedusa's famous line in *The Leopard*, 'If we want things to stay as they are, things will have to change', could be read as either positive and constructive or negative and threatening. Change was certainly very much part of the hospital's agenda at this time, as the 1993 annual report explained:

> As a result of the state government's decision in 1991 to maintain Fairfield Hospital as a viable clinical facility, a process of change was implemented to ensure that the hospital was better positioned to meet the future health care needs of Victoria.

The key elements of the health care process were:
1. A central Steering Committee to oversee the implementation process.
2. An internal efficiency review process in most hospital departments.

As a result of the efficiency review process, a number of important changes were implemented, including:
1. A review of work practices leading to better staff utilisation.
2. The establishment of a ten bed Continuing Care Unit and C.T. Scanning Service.
3. The reconstruction of the Kitchen to facilitate a centralised food plating and dishwashing system.

The co-operation of staff, unions and the Department of Health & Community Services (DHSC) throughout this entire process is greatly appreciated. This process has put us in a good position to meet the budgetary constraints anticipated for the 1993/94 financial year, as well as providing a more efficient hospital with a wider range of clinical services.

We are pleased to welcome a number of new organisations onto our campus, including the Australian Institute of Environmental Health, the Victorian Community Health Standards Program, the Health Industry Training Board, Paramedical Software, Health Solutions Pty. Ltd., the VHA Cytomix Facility and the Positive Women's Group, all of which complement our expanding role in health care delivery.

One thing that had not changed for the better was the continuing depredations of the AIDS epidemic. In 1992/93, 124 new cases were seen at Fairfield, making a cumulative total of 716 cases. This confirmed the increase and stabilisation in the predicted annual incidence. The AIDS cases seen at Fairfield represented 88 per cent of all cases notified in Victoria. To June 1993 there had been 937 cases diagnosed in Victoria. Of notified cases in 1992/93, 84 per cent were homosexual or bisexual men, 8 per cent were acquired by heterosexual contact and 4 per cent by injecting drug use. Research suggested that there had been little change in the established prevalence of risk behaviours. In the same period, 232 people were diagnosed HIV antibody positive in Victoria. This was approximately 10 per cent less than the previous 12 months, but brought the cumulative number of HIV antibody positive individuals in Victoria to 3041 (30 per cent of whom had already progressed to AIDS). Homosexual or bisexual men represented 70 per cent of new HIV diagnosis, and 14 per cent were heterosexual. Injecting drug use as a possible risk behaviour for acquisition of HIV occurred in only 5 per cent of new diagnoses for 1992/93. Although numbers remained small, 7 of the 32 cases of heterosexually acquired HIV infection reported exposure with a partner overseas.

Despite the intense demands of HIV/AIDS and fierce budgetary restraints, there was a continuing commitment to develop the hospital's non

HIV/AIDS clinical and support services. A good example of this were developments within the Long-term Ventilation Unit. The activity of the unit had been steadily increasing, and the emphasis on care had evolved from a residential to a community focus. It became possible to provide long-term ventilation in a community setting for most patients in the program. This was achieved by providing comprehensive ventilation training for patients. In response to increasing demand from post-polio patients for rehabilitation assessment, Dr Peter Colville was appointed rehabilitation consultant to the unit.

Dr Alvis Kucers, the Director of Medical Services, took sabbatical leave in January 1993 to work on the fifth edition of his world-acclaimed textbook on antibiotics. He retired on completing his sabbatical. Dr Kucers had made a notable contribution to the growth of Fairfield as a centre of excellence in infectious diseases. Dr Robert Grogan was appointed as the new Director of Medical Services in March 1993. Another notable retirement at this time was that of Dr Noel Bennett, Director of Quarantine Services. Bennett had served the hospital with distinction for many years in a variety of senior clinical and administrative roles. His career was at times controversial, but no one ever doubted his dedication and commitment to the hospital.

The amalgamation of Fairfield Hospital laboratories into the integrated Victorian Infectious Diseases Reference Laboratories (VIDRL) in 1993 was a recognition of the expertise of the laboratories and the national and international reputation which they enjoyed. The VIDRL was officially opened by Dr Chris Brook, Director of Public Health, on 4 June 1993. The inaugural Director of the VIDRL was Dr Stephen Locarini. (Locarini was later also appointed Associate Professor in the Department of Microbiology at Monash University). The official responsibilities and research activities of the VIDRL were impressive. The 1993 annual report listed its major functions and responsibilities at the state level:

1. Mycobacterium Reference Laboratory
2. Microbiology Department
3. Haematology Department
4. Biochemistry Department
5. Biomedical Reference Laboratory
6. Viral Identification Laboratory
7. Victorian HIV Reference Laboratory
8. Viral Hepatitis Reference Laboratory
9. Antivirals Laboratory
10. Electron Microscopy
11. Molecular Microbiology
12. Infectious Diseases Serology Laboratory

It also houses the National Hepatitis Reference Laboratory and the National High Security Quarantine Laboratory. The VIDRL is a designated World Health Organisation Reference Centre, with the following responsibilities:

1. WHO Collaborating Centre for Virus Reference Research
2. WHO Collaborating Centre for Biosafety and Training
3. WHO Influenza Laboratory
4. WHO Western Pacific Regional Reference Laboratory for Diagnosis of Poliomyelitis

The VIDRL provides epidemiological data to the Department of Health and Community Services, Victoria, contributes data fortnightly on its positive viral diagnoses to the Communicable Diseases Intelligence (CDI) Bulletin in Canberra, and reports influenza virus activity directly to the WHO in Geneva.

A report on nursing in the 1993 annual report presents all that was best —and arguably all that was worst—in the 'cutting edge' of new managerial attitudes and development strategies. Entitled 'Meeting the Demand', it is worth quoting at length:

> The nursing division has been moving from a traditional centralised organisational structure, towards autonomous clinical units with a concomitant empowerment of the unit managers and their staff. Creativity is being encouraged and fostered among the staff in their continual striving for excellence of nursing care.
>
> Last year began with a vision. A vision that the nursing division at Fairfield Hospital will become an international centre of nursing excellence, with strengths in education, research and clinical practice. In the past we have been less than successful in informing health professionals, external to Fairfield, of our excellence in nursing practice and it is definitely time to do so.
>
> To enable this vision to become a reality a number of objectives have to be met and these are:–
> * to stimulate the nursing staff towards shared desired goals
> * building of trust
> * the decentralisation of nursing administration
> * for unit managers to be responsible for 24 hour staffing of their unit
> * to develop a resource driven model of nursing care delivery
> * *to right size the nursing workforce* [my emphasis]
> * to restructure the division
> * the empowerment of the unit manager
>
> The vision has two dimensions—the services provided to clients and the management and organisation of the nursing services. The vision is providing the stimulus to strive for excellence by challenging the staff to stretch for and to achieve shared goals . . . The charge nurses have responded enthusiastically and individual units are now engaged in developing and implementing different modalities of client care. Our major objective here is to deliver the highest standard of nursing care possible. The staff involved in ward based quality assurance programs to measure the achievement of this goal from many different aspects.

A number of new communication initiatives in 1993 included the publication of *Fairfield Echo*, a new and authoritative newsletter conceived and published by senior medical staff, and widely distributed to doctors and other interested persons around the state. The hospital also launched a telephone Health Information Advice Line on 9 September 1993. This service, which provided pre-recorded travel health and other infectious disease information was, at least in part, established in an effort to stave off the large number of information-request telephone calls, for which the hospital had allocated no staffing or funding. This new service was supported by associated community services announcements shown extensively on television over the summer holidays. Another important communication development was the establishment of the Victorian Infectious Diseases Information Service in November 1993. Initiated by the Medical Research Librarian, this service provided up-to-date information on infectious diseases to general practitioners.

Following a meeting at the Positive Living Centre in St Kilda on 1 October 1993, Fairfield established a clinical annexe at the centre to provide medical and allied health services closer to the area where a good many of the hospital's HIV/AIDS patients lived. This started on 11 November 1993. Another major expansion of the hospital's facilities in 1994 was the refurbishment of Ward 1. This ward, which had previously been a paediatric unit, was re-equipped to function as a 25-bed acute infectious diseases unit, and was officially opened by the Director of Disability Services, Des O'Shea, on 24 June 1994.

Fairfield also successfully tendered for the management of the Melbourne Sexual Health Centre in Swanston Street, Carlton. This centre provided the hospital with an additional site from which ambulatory services could be delivered in the future. As part of the process of upgrading its services Fairfield, in conjunction with Monash University, decided to appoint a Professor of Venereology. Funding for this position was to be provided by the Department of Health and Community Services as part of the winning tender bid but, as it transpired, no appointment was made.

The vision of Fairfield becoming a broadly based public health campus was given added impetus by the nature of the tenant organisations it attracted, as the 1994 annual report noted:

> Over the past two years, Fairfield Hospital has attracted a number of tenant organisations who provide health related services. The inclusion of these tenants within the infrastructure of the campus has seen the development of a rich professional network. The collaboration of the tenant organisations with the hospital and each other has contributed to the overall quality and diversity of programs within the public health sector. The hospital will continue to encour-

age and support these vital networks which will not only benefit the campus, but the health and well being of the community as a whole.

Department of Health and Community Services:
Children and Family Health Services
Contact Tracing Services
Radiation Laboratory

Research and Reference:
Macfarlane Burnet Centre for Medical Research
National Centre for Health Program Evaluation
National HIV Reference Laboratory

Education:
Centre for Social Health
Health Industry Training Board

Health Services or Health Services Management:
Fairfield Hospital Travel Clinic
International Projects Group
Health Solutions Pty Ltd
Paramedical Softwear (STOCCA)
VHA Cytomix
Victorian Community Health Accreditation and Standards Program

Health Professional Societies:
Australian Institute of Environmental Health (Victorian Division)
Melbourne Division of General Practice

Self-Help and Consumer Organisations:
Hepatitis C Support Group
Positive Women
Victorian Consumer Health Voice.

Whether or not one supported the multi-faceted public health scenario advanced by the Board and senior hospital administrators, it was clearly more than a pipe dream. If Fairfield could have attracted enough financially viable public health tenants to make it economically self-sufficient, it might have secured its future—and perhaps even the future of on-site clinical services.

As part of Fairfield's attempt to become a public health resource and more 'user friendly', early in 1994 the Board approved the creation of honorary affiliated GPs, who were to be granted a number of privileges when they referred patients to Fairfield. The first group of affiliates, recruited after widespread promotion within the medical profession, were formally 'inducted' at a special function on 22 September 1994. In another positive development, the Department of Health and Community Services awarded the hospital a contract to manage a tuberculosis service in the former Ward 22. Originally a

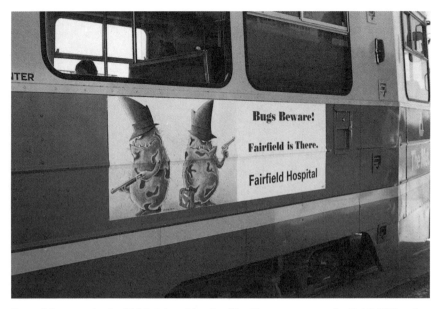

Part of the campaign in 1995, initated by Dr Allen Yung, to promote the Fairfield Travel Clinic.

six-month contract, this move proved so successful that it was soon extended to the end of 1995. It was generally felt that through strengthening the link between clinical and laboratory services based at Fairfield and the nursing contact tracers, a much better TB service was provided for Victoria.

The first year of 'casemix funding' was 1993/94. The formula for funding was centred upon a projection of length of patient hospital stay, based on the presenting/diagnosed illness—in other words, the government funded hospitals on the basis of predicted average length of stay for each illness. The hospital thus lost out if a misdiagnosis or some other factor led to a patient staying for longer than the 'average' time, and gained a financial advantage if the patient was discharged earlier than the 'average'. This new funding formula, introduced on 1 July 1993, incorporated a 10 per cent cut to Fairfield's budget (from $38.9 million to $35.1 million). Consequently, 48 staff received 'voluntary' departure packages during 1993/94.

Casemix funding was particularly harsh on a hospital such as Fairfield which specialised in complex and often intractable infectious diseases. Many of these diseases simply did not fit into the tidy patterns commonly experienced at other public hospitals. To establish an average length of stay for a tonsillectomy is a very different proposition from making the same calculation for a 'fever of unknown origin'. Casemix funding was by no means an ideal financial basis for an infectious diseases hospital and some Fairfield staff who were administering it believe that it sounded the death knoll for Fairfield's economic viability—or even near viability. In the 1994 annual report, Fairfield management stated that:

> In the first year of casemix funding we were very successful in achieving the $3.8 mill (10 per cent) budget cut applied by the Department of Health and Community Services (DH & CS), where our overall budget was reduced from $38.9m to $35.1m through application of the casemix funding formula. Our success in meeting this target is due to the many cost saving contributions made by all sections of the hospital, which is gratefully acknowledged. As most of the revenue needed to cover our costs comes from the number and types of patients treated under the casemix formula, it was important for us to maintain patient throughput, compared with the previous year. I am pleased to report that we were able to achieve this throughput objective in 1993–94.
>
> Furthermore, the success of our many marketing activities seem to be bearing fruit, and we have enjoyed high patient throughput over recent months. This will stand us in good stead in raising sufficient revenue in 1994–95 to meet our costs.

It may well be more accurate to say that the hospital was chasing its own tail. Any budget savings simply proved that previous budgets were far too high and could be further—much further—reduced. I would suggest that patient 'throughput' is no way to assess the quality, efficiency or financial needs of any clinical facility.

The Department of Health and Community Services (DH & CS), in June 1994, provided Fairfield with a grant to establish a Continuing Care Unit. The money enabled Fairfield to establish a statewide consultancy, support and education team in the area of palliative care for people living with HIV/AIDS. The money also meant that Fairfield could appoint a palliative care physician, a psychologist and a nurse to provide the service. Continuing care of a somewhat different sort was available when Fairfield's Multi-Faith Centre was finally constructed after several years of fund raising. This centre enabled the hospital to better meet the spiritual needs of its patients, staff and the broader community. It was officially opened at a ceremony on 25 July 1994 attended by leaders of a number of faiths represented in the community served by the hospital.

Through funds from the entrepreneurial education programs conducted by the Vivian Bullwinkel Education Centre, the hospital was able to extensively renovate the education centre. The hospital had begun marketing the centre and its education programs as part of the process of developing a major public health/infectious diseases education facility for the hospital and the state. The renovated building was opened by the Deputy Secretary of the DH & CS, Peter Allen, on behalf of the Minister for Community Services, Michael John, on 31 August 1994.

Since the establishment of the Fairfield Campus Information Network (FCIN) in 1991, the hospital's electronic information system now had 40 internal users and 202 external subscribers, who could gain access to Fairfield's extensive data files on infectious diseases. During 1993/94, the team of staff who operated FCIN developed a national electronic network called HealthNet Australia. This network was officially launched by Senator Peter Cook in Sydney on 9 September 1994 at the inaugural meeting of the National Health Industry Development Forum. This launch opened up Fairfield's data files to the world through the Internet, to which it was linked, and also brought data files from around the world back to Fairfield. Its success was recognised—and extended—by negotiations for the network to become the national electronic communications system for the Australian Hospitals Association.

In May, the hospital's marketing division sponsored the establishment of a Fairfield auxiliary called Faircarers, which amongst other things established an opportunity shop that was officially opened on 18 July 1994. The auxiliary also operated a patient services trolley to the wards. Both patients and staff had much cause to be grateful to the many friends of Fairfield who so generously contributed their time, talent and energy to Faircarers and its predecessors.

The hospital concluded negotiations with the MBCMR, in June 1994, for the centre to take a 40-year lease on the former Wards 15 and16. It planned to renovate the wards for use as a laboratory complex. Fairfield management were very pleased to have made this mutually beneficial arrangement, as it was recognised that 'The MBC is an important part of our campus, and its staff and services complement those provided by the hospital'.

As part of its educational and community health role, Fairfield published a wide range of literature available either free or by subscription service. By 1994 the following publications and pamphlets were available from the hospital at no charge: *Relatives and Friends Handbook; Patients Handbook; Information for Parent or Guardian of a Child Patient; Information re. Deceased Estates; Patients' Rights and Responsibilities*. Publications for sale included *Health Advice for Travellers; Through the Maze: Services for People with HIV/AIDS; Fairfield Hospital HIV Handbook: A Manual for Clinicians Working with HIV Infection*. Fairfield had always taken its educational and community health responsibilities seriously, and there can be no doubt that its publications played a significant role in improving knowledge about infectious disease among both the general public and health professionals. This commitment to education was reflected by the fact that La Trobe University joined the University of Melbourne and Monash University in affiliating with Fairfield in 1994, and that Deakin University and the Royal Melbourne Institute of Technology were also negotiating to affiliate.

On 2 December 1994 the *Age* published an article entitled 'Six Hospital Closures Mooted', in which a 'confidential Health Department document' was quoted as foreshadowing the closure of Fairfield and five other hospitals. The following month, the state government released a statement entitled 'Victoria's Health to 2050—Developing Melbourne's Hospital Network'. This statement, which outlined the problems in the hospital system and recommended some radical changes, led to the establishment of the Metropolitan Hospitals' Planning Board (MHPB). Established on 3 February 1995, it subsequently recommended the creation of seven hospital networks across Melbourne, as organisational vehicles for providing 'seamless' patient care closer to where people live. Fairfield was to be placed in the North Eastern Network, along with the Austin/Repatriation Medical Centre, Preston and Northcote Community Hospital, Mercy Hospital (the Mercy, however, was never a fully participating part of the network) and a proposed new community hospital at Epping. It was hoped that 'Within this framework there should be greater opportunities for sharing services and knowledge in providing improved health services in the north-east and in improving tertiary referral services'. Ominously, the MHPB proposed, in an *Interim Report* published on 30 April 1995, that Fairfield should merge with the Austin Repatriation Medical Centre.

Steve Dow, medical writer for the *Age*, wrote an article entitled 'Deadly Remedy' in April 1995. It reflected on the effect on CEO Chris Richards of the announcement by state government in March that it intended to establish an institute of forensic psychiatry on the hospital campus:

> For a hospital administrator who sees Fairfield becoming the 'CDC of the South'—emulating the prestigious Centres for Disease Control in Atlanta—it was a body blow. Government denials have disappeared. When the Kennett government proposed last month to build on the Fairfield site a forensic institute—a hospital for dangerously mentally ill prisoners—Mr Richards embraced the plan, even although the new buildings will compromise the tranquil AIDS garden. He saw it as a chance to keep Fairfield on site. But there has never been such a promise … Fairfield has had four directors of medicine since 1993 … Mr Richards plays down his differences with the medical staff as more philosophical. He wants a combined research–clinical service of international renown, and says the doctors are focussed only on hospital services. 'I've fought

for this dream all my time at Fairfield,' he says. 'It's a real chance for Melbourne to grab for something' [an obvious baited line for Kennett, who was keen to attract enterprises to Victoria]. A Kennett government in a generous mood might let the dream proceed, but if such an institute was to be allowed on the present site, it would probably be based on research, without a hospital. If the laboratories and the hospital stay together, they will probably be moved and fall under another hospital's control. Either way, Fairfield Hospital, as we know it, appears on the ebb.[9]

Some Fairfield staff would later allocate a good deal of the blame for the closure of Fairfield to Richards, but it should be noted that some of his management staff saw him as the first Executive Director to fully recognise that the Kennett government's hospital restructuring plans threatened the future not only of Fairfield but also of other public hospitals in Melbourne. Clearly Richards had a vision for the hospital that was not shared by many of its staff, but equally clearly his vision was based on the hospital continuing to exist— albeit in a radically altered, perhaps non-clinical, form.

Certainly, in the 1995 annual report Richards was still putting a strong case for the hospital's financial viability:

> At the conclusion of the year past, it is helpful to reflect on how we gave real meaning to the maxim of 'doing much more with much less'. It was indeed a year in which we were able to provide additional services to our patients from a reduced budget base.
>
> Fairfield has been successful in meeting a budget cut of approximately $3m, determined by the funding formula of the department of Health and Community Services.
>
> We can now proudly proclaim to our patients, the taxpayers and the government funder, that our level of patient services is higher than it was in the year before casemix was introduced (1992/93), with a fifth less funding allocation to achieve this end.

As well as highlighting the hospital's financial 'success', Richards continued to promote his vision, noting that 'During the year we welcomed two new tenant organisations onto the campus to join the growing number of agencies that value the prospect of creating a public health campus on our site'. In his efforts to ensure that Fairfield had some sort of future Richards even managed to put a positive spin on the government's plan, announced in March 1995, to establish an institute of forensic psychiatry (sometimes described as a hospital for the criminally insane) in the hospital grounds. The hospital, Richards wrote:

> has assessed this initiative to ensure that it can be achieved without compromising our long standing function as an infectious diseases hospital, and the planning process is now well underway. A number of buildings in the southern annexe are

affected, and several services will be relocated to under-utilised buildings else-where on site. We are now looking forward to having this new facility interacting co-operatively with Fairfield and our tenants.

Steve Dow was particularly well informed regarding the state of play in respect to Fairfield's future. Writing in the *Age* on 18 May 1995 under the headline 'AIDS group warns on Fairfield closure', he explained the hospital's position:

> AIDS lobbyists are seeking a state government assurance that it will save Fairfield hospital amid new fears it could close within months rather than years.
>
> Well-placed sources say the government is investigating moving AIDS services elsewhere within months rather than years.
>
> It is believed the number of beds for HIV patients at the Alfred hospital may be increased. 'There won't be a hospital at Fairfield in two years,' one source said.
>
> The Health Department was carrying out a 'white-anting exercise' to 'dismantle the place as soon as possible'. Fairfield's marketing division was winding up and bed occupancy was below 70 per cent 'It's a self-fulfilling prophecy,' the source said.
>
> In its bid to save Fairfield the Victorian Aids Council will meet the Health Minister's parliamentary secretary, Dr Dennis Napthine, on Monday and will hold a public meeting at the hospital tonight. The council's president, Mr Bradley Engelmann, said the council was sceptical about the government's intentions. 'Personally I do think they have an agenda for the site . . . This might

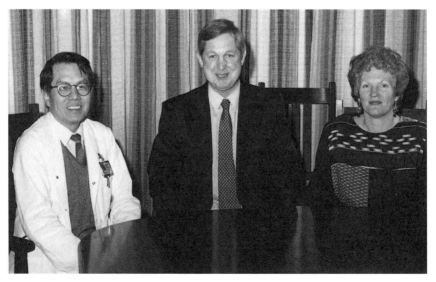

Senior hospital staff in about 1995: Dr Allen Yung, Director of Medical Services (left); Chris Richards, Chief Executive Officer; Peg Higginbottom, Director of Nursing.

include new psychiatric facilities to accompany a forensic psychiatry unit to be
built at Fairfield this year,' he said.

Last month the Metropolitan Hospital's Planning Board proposed in a preliminary report that Fairfield merge with the Austin–Repatriation Medical
Centre.

But the chief executive of the Austin–Repat, Dr Michael Stanford, previously
said Fairfield could not be moved for at least five years because it would take at
least that long for building to begin at the former Heidleberg Repatriation
Hospital site.

Another senior Aids group figure said there was concern that the promise of
a five-year delay was a 'whitewash'. With the new super-hospital boards due to
be appointed on 1 July, no guarantees could be given. The Fairfield management
is working to ensure that at least the laboratories stay on the site.

Despite the dramatic style, the content of this report was to prove largely
correct and the analysis of the situation by 'well-placed sources' within gay
organisations was remarkably accurate. A good many rumours about the
future of Fairfield were flying around at this time—rumours fuelled by the
increased sympathy of MHPB to arguments favouring the closure of Fairfield. Fairfield and other 'at risk' public hospitals were feeling isolated and
vulnerable. This feeling was heightened by the fact that the individual boards
of management that had for so long played such a crucial role in hospital
development and administration in Victoria's public hospital network were
being phased out as part of the 'rationalisation' and streamlining of the hospital system.

The internal and external divisions, insecurities and fears for the future
permeating the hospital community at this time were well explored—and
perhaps exacerbated—by an article in the *Age* on 19 May, entitled 'Fairfield
chiefs betrayed us: AIDS groups':

> AIDS lobbyist last night slammed Fairfield Hospital management, claiming it
> had betrayed them by allegedly calling for the hospital to close.
>
> Victorian AIDS Council representatives last night condemned Fairfield's
> chief executive, Chris Richards, for allegedly telling the Metropolitan Hospitals
> Planning Board in a meeting on Wednesday night that Fairfield should be
> quickly transferred to the Austin–Repatriation Medical Centre at Heidelberg.
>
> The council's support program manager, Ms Vicki King, declared at a public
> meeting at Fairfield last night that Richards 'didn't have any bloody right to
> represent that view to the committee'.

The president of the Australian Federation of Aids Organisations, Tony
Keenan, and a Fairfield board member, David Menadue, publicly supported
King's statement. Richards had not been available for comment that week,
but a Fairfield spokeswoman had said that Fairfield management believed 'the

end' had come for the hospital. This, the *Age* reported, was despite the Board's earlier call to retain Fairfield:

> On 30 April the planning board's preliminary report proposed that Fairfield merge with the Austin–Repatriation centre, signalling that it should move to the Heidelberg campus.
>
> An angry crowd meeting in Fairfield's recreation hall last night called for:
> • An assurance from the State government and the Austin–Repatriation centre that HIV services will remain on the Fairfield campus.
> • Maintenance of all HIV services, buildings and infrastructure.
> • The Victorian Infectious Diseases Laboratory remain on the site.
> • An HIV care committee to be set up from 1 July with members of HIV community groups.
> • Clinical services trials and research be kept together.
> • Extra HIV beds to be made available at the Alfred Hospital, but not at Fairfield's expense.
>
> Dr Anne Mijch said the medical staff supported a merger with the Austin centre because otherwise Fairfield would remain weak and relatively expensive.
>
> She said HIV beds would be better maintained at Fairfield.
>
> However, the medical staff's submission to the planning board made the future location negotiable.
>
> An HIV patient said the community should expect nothing less than Fairfield.
>
> 'Closing this hospital is a bad management that we'll pay for in the future,' he said, 'and we have already bloody paid enough.'
>
> The chief executive of the Austin–Repatriation centre, Mr Michael Stanford, said it would be three or four years before Fairfield could move to Heidelberg.

It was clear that the decision to close Fairfield had been made, and all that remained to be decided was the timing of its closure.

The Health Services Union of Australia, Victoria No. 1 Branch published an Impact Assessment of the Phase 1 Report of the Metropolitan Hospitals Planning Board in July 1995. This commented tersely on the MHPB proposals for Fairfield: 'Transfer of clinical services to other sites within the North East Network—closure implied. Decision re non-clinical services to be decided by H&CS (libraries, laboratories). No mention of McFarlane Burnet Centre.' Its conclusion reflected the concerns of many people in the community about changes being made to the Victorian hospital system:

> The Reports of the Metropolitan Hospital Planning Board are long on rhetoric and assertions, but short on reasoning and relevant data. The Board has delivered what the Government asked for—a plan to amalgamate and rationalise public hospital services. The restructuring of the acute care hospital system which is proposed will have significant effects on the delivery of services and the viability of some hospitals, with the overall bed numbers falling. Staffing levels will

also fall. The industrial relations implications of the proposed changes are ignored by the MHPB . . . The Reports, of course, were not designed to stand up to detailed scrutiny, but to serve a political purpose in delivering a series of justifications for the direction in which the Victorian government had already decided to move in downgrading Victoria's public health system.[10]

For Fairfield Hospital, the end came quickly—faster than even the most pessimistic of hospital staff expected. Even after the MHPB reports which recommended the closure appeared, there were some grounds for optimism —after all, Fairfield had been threatened by closure many times in its history and had survived, and memories of the successful defence of the hospital earlier in the decade were still fresh in people's minds. Senior administrators had gone on record as saying that it would take three to four years to close the hospital, and such a time span made sense in terms of the complex and very sensitive nature of such a move. Given such a delay, there was always the possibility that the situation could alter—a change of government, for example—and the hospital might once again win an unlikely last-minute reprieve.

In the event, the hospital not only failed to win a reprieve but was in fact closed by the middle of 1996. There were many reasons why the closure took place and why it occurred so quickly. In the first place, one should note that staff had barely recovered from the fiercely fought campaign that they and the hospital's community-based supporters had waged only a few years before. Thus, although the staff fought valiantly through various forms of union-organised activities—including round-the-clock picketing—there was a sense that this was a fight that had to be made but which was unlikely to save the hospital. The government under Premier Kennett was committed to radical-conservative 'economic rationalist' theories and, moreover, prided itself on making decisions swiftly and acting immediately without giving much, if any, thought to community concerns or protests.

It is also widely held that the campaign to save the hospital was damaged by the withdrawal of support from the well-organised and influential Victorian AIDS Council. Some senior union officers believe that this withdrawal of support for the continuation of the hospital, particularly in the light of the crucial part AIDS organisations had played in the 1991 campaign, effectively sealed the hospital's fate. While not wishing to discount the importance of the AIDS Council's decision, it is fanciful to imagine that its support could have swung the balance and saved the hospital. In truth, once the Liberal government had decided to close Fairfield, there was only an extremely remote chance that it could be saved. The leaders of the AIDS Council and of other patient representative groups associated with the hospital had an obligation to

promote the best interests of their members and those whom they represented. When it became obvious that the closure of Fairfield was
a 'done deal', in *real politik* terms these organisations were duty bound to cut
their losses and try to win the best possible outcome for their members.

With closure looming, Fairfield's final months were a time of great
bitterness and sadness. Fierce divisions and ill-feelings came to a head among
the staff. Unionised workers and most of the medical staff, fighting tenaciously
to save Fairfield, often harboured intense antipathy towards those in hospital
management who were seen—not always fairly—as complicit in the closure
of the hospital. Ill-feeling within the hospital was compounded by union
cleaning bans and other militant industrial actions which made the hospital's
last weeks chaotic and fraught and which, ironically, may have led to the hospital closing a few days earlier than had been planned.

Some of the bitterness and anger of Fairfield's last days might have been
mitigated if those staff members who were losing their jobs had been given a
fair and reasonable financial settlement. The parsimony and injustice of the
redundancy packages that staff were forced to accept rubbed salt on open
wounds. Of particular concern to staff was the iniquitous division of redundancy packages according to age. Workers under 55 who were made redundant due to the closure of the hospital received a lump sum of $10 000 and
two weeks of pay for each year of continuous service, up to a specific number
of years. Workers who were over 55, on the other hand, were eligible for only
$5000 and one week of pay for each year of service, also up to a specific
number of years. The redundancy payment for those under 55 was far from
handsome, but the treatment of workers over the age of 55—who would find
it more difficult to get work—was scandalous.

On Sunday 12 May 1996, Dr A. Murray Sandland gave a farewell speech
to a large gathering of Fairfield staff, past and present, and supporters of the
hospital. Because there was no public address system, Dr Sandland felt con-
strained to give an abbreviated version of the speech he had prepared. What
follows is the whole of the speech he planned. His words form a fitting conclusion to this study of a hospital which generations of Victorians had come
to trust and respect.

> The natural person to have been asked to speak at the gathering would have
> been Dr Allen Yung, our Chief of Medicine, who has been a staff member for 33
> years. As he is in the early stages of convalescence after surgery the task fell to
> me. As I have been a staff member for just over 30 years, I too feel deeply at this
> time, and I speak as current Chair of the Medical Staff.
>
> I would like to hang my thoughts this afternoon on three words.

1. Anger

My first word may not be universally popular for various reasons at a gathering like this. I deal with it first, but I believe it must be dealt with if we are to be honest about why we are here today.

The word is Anger.

(a) Anger at the dismemberment of a centre of excellence
   – services going to various places
   – decisions about where our laboratories will go and whether they will all move ion one direction not yet made, let alone whether they will go with one of the major services.

(b) Anger that it has become easier and easier to close us
   – lack of government commitment
   – successive budget cuts

(c) Anger at a planning process which largely ignored the insights of our vastly experienced staff.

   A tender process, which though supposedly open was clearly intended to divide the clinical services.

(d) Anger at the way our network handled the process, treating us as political liabilities, at odds with their business interests, anxious to close down clinical services as early as possible, using the excuse of union bans to achieve this.

   (When Fairfield had its own board, the monthly meetings were often extremely tense affairs. Dr Allen Yung once told the board in my presence that attending board meetings was the most unpleasant part of his job at Fairfield. But at least they had to listen to clinical concerns. We have no direct input into network board deliberations. I don't even know what the chair looks like. What has the network known of us? And why have they refused permission repeatedly to us to talk to the media about things in which hospital doctors and scientists have more experience than similar people from other institutions.)

(e) Anger about our final weeks here. This anger is a complicated one.
   – Our final days at the hospital have been more unpleasant than they need have been. We were not allowed to admit patients for several periods before in-patient services finally closed.
   – Cleaning has become a real problem.
   – The loss of a social focus, when there were no longer cafeteria meals.
   – Staff solidarity has been shattered.
   – Alternative places have received patients, even less ready for them than they would have been by May 31st let alone June 30th.

   But this anger is two-sided: while angry that union workers have imposed these things on us, this blends with an anger *shared* with them, with such obvious inequities in payouts for people who will have no jobs after the closure.

   So much for anger, now let us soften it and talk about.

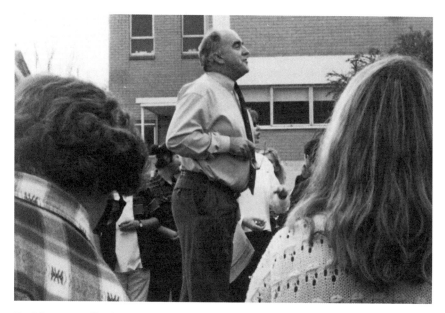

Dr Murray Sandland speaks to the farewell gathering in May 1996.

2. *Sorrow*
(a) Sorrow for loss of physical surrounding, not only precious in themselves, but also because they have allowed us to practice the particular type of healing art for which this place is famous.
   - the gardens
   - the peacocks
   - the chapel—only open 2 years but meaning much to many staff and patients.
(b) Sorrow for loss of clinical interactions with laboratories.
(c) Sorrow at saying goodbye to colleagues of all sorts.
   - the attrition over some years
   - those we say goodbye to now or very shortly
   - those who won't have jobs, or whose jobs will be very different
   - those whom we have relied on, in many areas different from ours, so that all are helped to work better.
(d) Sorrow for our patients
   - who are already starting to encounter the real world of big public hospitals.
   - Here there has usually been no problem in finding a bed for an admission, and on discharge the ability to delay going home for a day or two, to get on one's feet.

(e) Finally Sorrow for Victoria and Beyond.
  - the loss of a central focus of clinical expertise in infectious diseases.
  - cutting edge lab. work and research
  - good teaching
  - and an information service for all who seek it whether within or outside Victoria.

And so sorrow in its turn gives way to—

3. *Pride*

As we remember what we have been, and in some senses still are

(a) Pride in our Caring Tradition
  Being prepared to put ourselves at risk throughout the period for some risky diseases, with no foolproof protection or treatment.
  - nurses ostracised in 30s, 40s who care for polio patients
  - our readiness to dialyse Hepatitis B carriers, when other hospitals didn't wish to treat them
  - caring for minority groups with Hepatitis B in the 70s meaning we were largely unfazed when these same groups turned up in the 80s with AIDS
  - our care of leprosy sufferers
  - our 'iron lung' ward.

(b) Pride in the family atmosphere—people working to one end, dented but not destroyed by professional jealousies or accountant administrators.

(c) Pride in our Laboratories—not just service institutions but the cutting edge of new techniques meeting challenges in identification of new infection agents.

(d) Pride in our Teaching of doctors, nurses and scientists so that there is a bit of Fairfield not only in most places of this continent, but in a lot of overseas countries.

(e) Pride in our deliberate contributions to infectious diseases internationally
  - supplying personnel overseeing widespread eradication of smallpox-polio
  - our World Health Organisation reference labs
  - the great antibiotics textbook [by] Kucers and Bennett, launched from here.

(f) Pride in Clinical Research of a high standard
  - despite vastly depleted infrastructure
  - what other hospital of this size has been able to make such a contribution to so many drug trials? Not many I think.

(g) Pride even in our last days
  - in the need for volunteers who have worked for many weeks on behalf of us and our patients
  - in all staff who performed extra duties so we could keep looking after patients as long as possible
  - in so many who doggedly stuck to Fairfield, even knowing it ultimately had no future, steadfastly ignoring the blandishments of other jobs or departure packages which, if taken would have rendered the hospital inoperable months ago.

The government may be proud that they have closed this place. Surely we should be proud, that, against the odds, we kept such a unique institution alive and as well as possible for 93 years. And to that all staff past and present have contributed.

I don't think people stop being Fairfield people when our day-to-day work here ceases. Many of you have not worked here for some years, in some cases many years, but still you have been able to bask in the community esteem that this hospital has enjoyed through its existence, and you have carried its traditions and insights into new jobs, or into retirement.

For those who have been staff members right up to the fall of the auctioneer's hammer, it is wonderful for us to know that we are highly esteemed not only by Victorians but by the International Community. The international letter writers, who annoyed Mrs Tehan [Minister for Health] so much, needed little or no prompting to acknowledge Fairfield's place in the wider picture.

So let us not live consumed by anger or sorrow, but proud of what we have given, with an assurance that it will remain relevant in whatever new spheres we find ourselves.

May God bless us all.

Keep the Spirit of Fairfield alive.[11]

The last seven AIDS patients were transferred from Fairfield on the day after the staff gathering—13 May 1996. The five remaining patients—all long-term patients in the respiratory unit—were transferred to other hospitals within the next few days . . .

APPENDICES

1 Chronology

2 Office-holders

3 Nursing Awards 1963–1989

4 Treatment Statistics
   Admissions/Discharges 1914–1996
   Major Diseases 1914–1936

5 Aims and Objectives

6 Organisational Structure 1995/96

7 Fairfield's Legacy, the Victorian Infectious Diseases
   Reference Laboratory

APPENDIX 1
Chronology

1789   Smallpox first recorded among Australian Aborigines.

1804   *Sydney Gazette* (14 October) published 'General Observations of the Smallpox' by Principal Surgeon Thomas Jamison. This was the colony's first medical treatise.

1826   Pierre Bretonneau describes and names diphtheria.

1832   Australia's first *Quarantine Act* passed.

1836   First hospital opened in Melbourne.

1838   First trained nurses in Australia—five nuns of the Sisterhood of Charity —arrive in Australia from Ireland and begin work at the Parramatta female convict factory.

1840   *A Familiar Treatise on the Diseases of the Eye*, by Robert Porter Welch, published—the first medical textbook to be separately printed and published in Australia.

1841   *Paper on the Present Epidemic of Scarlatina* by William Bland. A report on the colony's first scarlet fever epidemic.

1846   Port Phillip Medical Association founded—the first Australian medical society.

1847   Ether anaesthesia used for the first time in Australia (by Dr William Pugh of Launceston).

1848   Yarra Bend Lunatic Asylum opened.

1848   Melbourne Hospital opened.

1850   First recorded incidence of measles in Australia, in Victoria.

1852   The migrant ship *Ticonderoga* arrived at Hobson's Bay, Port Phillip. During the voyage 168 of her 814 passengers died of typhus.

1854   Victoria's first Public *Health Act* passed—establishing Central Board of Health.

1856   Lying-in Hospital (later Royal Women's Hospital) opened.

1857   Discovery of leprosy at Castlemaine, Victoria, created widespread fear of an epidemic.

1858   First recorded incidence of diphtheria on mainland Australia.

1859   509 Victorians die from diphtheria and croup. Professional training for nurses began with a formal midwifery training program at the Melbourne Lying-In Hospital.

1862   Medical School established at the University of Melbourne; the first students were enrolled in 1863.

1864	The Victorian government introduced compulsory registration of all charities, including public hospitals.
1869	Victorian Central Board of Health recommends the establishment of a contagious diseases hospital in Melbourne; Eye and Ear Hospital opened; Homeopathic Hospital (later Prince Henry's) opened.
1870	Children's Hospital opened.
1871	Alfred Hospital opened.
1872	Victorian government appoints a Royal Commission to inquire into all aspects of diphtheria.
1873	Inebriate Retreat, Merri Creek, opened.
1874	Victorian Central Board of Health in its fifteenth Annual Report notes that Victorian Government intended to make provision for the establishment of an infectious diseases hospital. Victorian *Compulsory Vaccination Act* requires that all children be vaccinated against smallpox within six months of birth.
1875	Australian Health Society founded in Melbourne; it pioneered health education through public lectures, classes and publications such as *The Sanitary Alphabet*.
1876	Victoria's highest scarlet fever mortality figures: 2240 deaths. In Brisbane, Dr Joseph Bancroft discovered the cause of filariasis (sometimes called elephantiasis).
1879	The Victorian Aborigines Board reported that the Aboriginal population of Victoria was declining rapidly due to 'lung disease' and other medical conditions. The report concluded that unhealthy living conditions were responsible for the terrible health and high mortality rates, and called for improved diet, accommodation and hygiene.
1882	Austin Hospital for Incurables opened. Williamstown Sanatorium built to house smallpox sufferers from Melbourne.
1887	First meeting of the St John Ambulance Association held in Melbourne, and an Ambulance Brigade established soon after.
1890	New *Public Health Act* abolished Central Board of Health and established a nine-member Board of Public Health and a Department of Health, under a Minister. D. A. Gresswell (City of Melbourne Health Officer and, from 1894, Chairman of the Board of Public Health) published *Report on the Sanitary Conditions of Melbourne*, stressing the desperate need for an infectious diseases hospital in Melbourne. 1031 Victorians die from diphtheria. Diphtheria antitoxin developed.
1893	St Vincent's Hospital opened. Perspective for a proposed infectious diseases hospital prepared by architects Wharton Down and Gibbons. Anti-diphtheria serum developed by Emil Behring.
1896	Diphtheria antitoxin first used in Victoria at the Children's Hospital. Queen Victoria Memorial Hospital for Women and Children opened in Melbourne.
1897	Queen Victoria's Diamond Jubilee. Mayor of Melbourne, Councillor Strong, convenes a meeting to set up an infectious diseases hospital in Melbourne. Government granted fifteen acres on Yarra Bend for the establishment of a Fever Hospital.

1899	Australasian Trained Nurses Association founded in Sydney; Victoria the only state not to form a branch.
1900	Design of Queen's Memorial Hospital buildings completed, and work starts on building. First case of plague reported in Melbourne. Bubonic plague reported in Adelaide, and 103 people died of plague in Sydney.
1901	Queen's Memorial Hospital buildings completed. Victorian Trained Nurses Association formed in Melbourne.
1902	John Ashburton Thompson demonstrated how plague is transmitted and outlined measures for controlling its spread.
1904	Queen's Memorial Hospital [here under Fairfield] opened on 1 October.
1905	Thomas Lane Bancroft discovered that the organism of dengue fever was carried by mosquitoes.
1907	Pirquet devises a method for diagnosing tuberculosis. C. Ross Harrison develops tissue culture techniques.
1908	Australian Institute of Tropical Medicine established at Townsville, a joint enterprise by the Commonwealth and Queensland governments and the universities of Adelaide, Melbourne and Sydney. Commonwealth Quarantine Service established as part of the Trade and Customs Department.
1909	E. M. Walker appointed Matron of Fairfield. Scarlet Fever epidemic in Melbourne.
1910	Dr F. V. Scholes appointed Medical Superintendent of Fairfield.
1911	Victorian Bush Nursing Association formed.
1912	Public Inquiry into the running of Fairfield.
1913	Bela Schick discovered test for immunity from diphtheria.
1914	Act of Parliament provides for a Board of Management for Fairfield.
1916	New administration building, two new ward pavilions for Fairfield. *Venereal Diseases Act* passed. Commonwealth Serum Laboratories and Walter and Eliza Hall Institute established in Melbourne.
1918	Fairfield gazetted to care for infantile paralysis patients.
1919	New *Health Act* passed—Board of Public Health abolished and Commission of Public Health established. Act consolidated all existing *Health Acts* and incorporated further provisions from English Health Acts. Influenza epidemic 1919 ('Spanish flu' killed at least 20 million people from 1918 to spring 1919 in Europe, America and India).
1921	Eight cases of smallpox in Victoria. Commonwealth Health Department established.
1922	Two new ward pavilions for measles patients and a new brick store opened.
1924	Nurses Home (Yarra House) expanded to the south.
1927	15 cases of poliomyelitis in Victoria (eight deaths); Philip Drinker invents iron lung. Scarlet fever antitoxin introduced.
1928	156 cases of poliomyelitis in Victoria (25 deaths).
1929	Agnes McIntyre from St Thomas's Hospital in London became Australia's first almoner, at Melbourne Hospital (now Royal Melbourne Hospital).
1930	Association of Physicians of Australia and New Zealand formed.

1932   Nurses Home expanded.

1933   Influenza virus identified.

1934   Alexander Fleming and G. F. Petrie published *Recent Advances in Vaccine and Serum Therapy*.

1936   Fairfield purchased a Drinker Respirator. Commonwealth Government established the National Health and Medical Research Council.

1937   Epidemic of poliomyelitis began in southern suburbs of Melbourne, later spreading to all parts of Victoria. Government appointed a Consultative Council for Poliomyelitis. Commonwealth *Medical Research Endowment Act* made provision for a national research endowment fund.

1938   *National Health and Pensions Act* passed, establishing a contributory scheme of social security insurance including 'free' medical treatment, medicines and certain appliances. Association of Physicians of Australasia and New Zealand renamed Royal Australian College of Physicians. Australian Red Cross Society established a blood transfusion service.

1940   Fairfield became a training school for nurses. Australian scientist Howard Florey, whilst at Oxford, developed penicillin for medical use.

1943   *Ministry of Health Act* introduced into Parliament. Outbreak of typhoid fever caused by contaminated milk, and Fairfield treated 124 patients. First Nurse Graduation Ceremony held at Fairfield. Dr C. Swan of Adelaide discovered the link between deafness in children and maternal rubella infection during pregnancy; Commonwealth Serum Laboratories began producing penicillin in commercial quantities, and Australia became the first country to make penicillin commercially available for civilians.

1944   *Ministry of Health Act* came into operation, with all state medical services brought under one control and the Department of Health responsible for administering all health-related legislation. Federal Labor Government passed *Pharmaceutical Benefits Act*, providing free medicines, materials and appliances when prescribed by a doctor on a government form.

1945   Under the terms of the *Hospital Benefits Act* the Commonwealth agreed to pay six shillings per day for each patient occupying a public hospital bed, provided that charges in public wards were waived—this was the start of Commonwealth funding of institutional care on a national basis. Federal *Tuberculosis Act* passed. Australian Institute of Hospital Administrators established (later the Australian College of Health Service Administrators).

1946   Dr F. M. Burnet, later Sir Macfarlane Burnet, appointed Consultant Epidemiologist at Fairfield.

1947   The British Medical Association in Australia (now Australian Medical Association) rejected Federal Labor Party invitation to consider a national medical service as 'being invited to indulge in consideration of professional euthanasia'; medical practitioners refused to co-operate when the Federal Parliament passed a new *Pharmaceutical Benefits Act*. Federal *World Health Organisation Act* committed Australia to the constitution of the World Health Organisation.

1948   Dr H. McLorinan appointed Medical Superintendent of Fairfield. Australian Post-Graduate Federation in Medicine founded. New *Tuberculosis Act* passed, the 1945 Act having proven ineffective. Federal Labor Government passed the *National Health Service Act*, giving the Commonwealth a wide range of powers and control over health facilities and services.

1949   F. V. C. Scholes' block constructed at Fairfield. Fairhaven Women's Clinic closed. Commonwealth Institute of Child Health established. College of Nursing, Australia founded.

1950   Small laboratory established at Fairfield by Sir Macfarlane Burnet. Plans for national health scheme, based on voluntary insurance, announced by the Menzies Government.

1951   Victorian Hospitals and Charities Commission established Australia's first nurse-aide training school. Commonwealth introduced Pensioner Medical Service, which paid general practitioner fees for aged, invalid, widow, service pensioners, tuberculosis allowance recipients and their dependants. Korean haemorrhagic fever (Seoul hantavirus) first recorded.

1952   Commonwealth hospital benefits scheme established.

1953   Fairfield the first infectious diseases hospital to allow patient visiting. Introduction of Triple Antigen. Dengue and Argentine haemorrhagic fevers first recorded. *National Health Act* passed, repealing the Labor Government's *National Health Service Act*. Commonwealth medical benefits scheme started, with benefits paid only to contributors to voluntary medical insurance funds.

1954   *Infectious Diseases Hospital Act* came into operation: municipal councils were no longer required to contribute to the funds of the hospital and the government assuming full financial responsibility through the Hospitals and Charities Fund. Queen's Memorial Infectious Diseases Hospital was officially renamed Fairfield Hospital (the hospital had used that name since 1948).

1955   Matron Burbidge awarded Order of the British Empire Medal.

1956   Sir Albert Coates elected Chairman of Board of Management. Commonwealth Serum Laboratories started producing Salk vaccine to combat poliomyelitis infections, with Fairfield selected to test its safety. Kyasanur Forest disease (a tick-transmitted virus disease) first recorded. Charges for public ward accommodation introduced by all states except Queensland.

1957   The Asian flu epidemic in July–August, with 672 cases attributable to the epidemic admitted to Fairfield; 376 had pneumonia and there were 38 deaths. This epidemic was soon followed by epidemics of viral meningitis and infectious hepatitis; A. B. Sabin in the United States produced an oral polio vaccine.

1958   National Biological Standards Laboratory established, to test drugs for purity and potency and to formulate standards for therapeutic goods and their production.

1959   Sabin published results of his live attenuated polio vaccine tests. O'nyong nyong fever (similar to dengue fever) first recorded.

1960	Sir Macfarlane Burnet (with Sir Peter Medawar) won the Nobel Prize. Bolivian haemorragic fever first recorded.
1961	Dr J. A. Forbes appointed Medical Superintendent. Australian Medical Association registered as a corporate body.
1963	Coates Block constructed. Last diphtheria death at Fairfield.
1964	World Health Organisation designated Fairfield laboratory as Oceanic Regions Reference Centre for Enteroviruses and Respiratory Viruses.
1966	Live virus vaccine for rubella developed by Harry Meyer and Paul Parman.
1967	Sabin oral poliomyelitis vaccine programme introduced in Australia. Marburg disease first recorded.
1968	Major epidemic of Hong Kong flu in Melbourne, which quickly spread throughout Australia. M. Arnstein developed a vaccine against meningitis.
1969	Lassa fever first recorded.
1970	Human toxoplasmosis first recorded.
1975	Lyme disease first recorded.
1976	29 people died of 'mystery' disease (later named Legionnaire's disease) at a meeting of the American Legion in Philadelphia. Ebola fever first recorded.
1977	Two homosexual men in San Francisco died of Kaposi's sarcoma— thought to have been the first victims of AIDS. Adult T-cell leukemia and Rift Valley fever first recorded.
1978	Vivian Bullwinkel Education Centre built. Federal government decided to build National High Security Quarantine Unit at Fairfield, in response to the increasing danger posed by imported viral haemorrhagic fevers.
1980	Vaccine for hepatitis B tested in the United States.
1981	HIV/AIDS (Acquired Immune Deficiency Syndrome) epidemic first recognised by US Centres for Disease Control.
1982	Haemophilia-associated AIDS first reported in the United States. Opening of National High Security Quarantine Unit at Fairfield.
1983	Research Centre at Fairfield established. Researchers at the US National Cancer Institute and at the Pasteur Institute in France isolated the virus thought to cause AIDS, which became known as the HIV virus.
1986	Fairfield Research Centre renamed Macfarlane Burnet Centre for Medical Research. (incorporated as a separate legal entity in 1989).
1993	Amalgamation of Fairfield laboratories into the integrated Victorian Infectious Diseases Reference Laboratories. Hantavirus pulmonary syndrome first recorded.
1994	Fairfield Hospital, Ward 1, converted from paediatric unit into a 25-bed acute infectious diseases unit.
1996	(30 June) Fairfield Hospital closed.

APPENDIX 2
Office-holders

Chairpersons of the Board

1904	Cr Sir Malcolm D. McEacharn
1904–15	Alderman W. Strong
1915–17	Cr T. Smith
1917–19	Cr B. J. Ferdinado
1919–22	Cr W. E. Cash
1922–23	Dr A. Jeffreys-Wood
1923–24	Cr E. Coulson
1924–28	Sir George Cuscaden MD
1928–29	Cr A. G. Proudfoot
1929–31	Dr J. Newman-Morris
1931–36	The Hon J. G. Membrey
1936–39	Cr G. R. A. Beardsworth
1939–41	Cr E. H. Hester
1941–45	The Hon Sir Herbert H. Olney
1945–46	Cr H. C. Edwards
1946–49	Mr M. Parker
1949–50	Cr N. G. Ibbott
1950–53	Mr R. Ivey
1953–56	The Hon A. E. Shepherd MLA
1956–73	Sir Alfred Coates
1973–75	Mr E. D. Oates
1975–77	Mr R. C. Allison
1977–79	Cr R. W. Gleeson
1979–81	Mr P. P. Gill
1981–82	Dr I. A. G. Brand AM (Administrator)
1982–84	Dr I. A. G. Brand AM
1984–87	Miss M. A. H. Taylor AM
1987–90	The Hon G. P. Connard MLC
1990–92	Professor N. F. Mills AC
1992–94	Mr A. H. Gray
1994–95	Professor A. C. L. Clark AM

Honorary Life Governors

Mr M. Becker
Mr J. Blom
Mrs M. Brierly
Miss M. Coates
Mr M. Herman
Mr R. Hooper
Mrs E. Joyce
Mrs B. Koren
Professor N. Millis
Mrs B. Nagle
Mr J. Parkes
Mrs A. Slater
Mrs L. Sherring
Mrs J. Shillitoe
Lady Marigold Southey
Ms M. Taylor
Mr H. Weatherley

Medical Superintendents/Directors of Medical Services

Medical Superintendents

1904–05	Dr S. H. Allen
1906	Drs P. C. Boyd, F. H. Makin and A. Haynes
1907	Dr M. K. Moss
1908	Dr C. V. Mackay
1909	Dr H. J. Gray
1910–48	Dr F. V. Scholes
1948–60	Dr H. McLorinan
1961–78	Dr J. A. Forbes

Medical Director and Chief Executive Officer

1979–81	Dr N. McKenzie Bennett

Director of Medical Services

1981–93	Dr A. Kucers
1993–94	Dr R. Grogan
1994	Dr A. Yung (Acting)
1994–96	Dr H. Wellington

Senior Executives

Manager/Secretary

1904	Mr G. V. Sylvester
1905–06	Mr A. U. Ellis
1907–14	Mr H. Crosbie
1915–38	Mr A. A. Marsden
1939–49	Mr N. W. Neep
1950–78	Mr B. D. Dynon

Administrator

1981–82 (17.2.81–10.3.82)	Dr I. A. G. Brand

Executive Directors

1981–85	Mr G. Houghton
1985–88	Mr W. R. Phillips
1988–96	Mr C. F. Richards

Matrons/Directors of Nursing

Matrons

1904–06	Miss E. A. Conyers
1907	Miss R. L. Shappere / Miss A. M. Jenkins
1908	Miss A. M. Jenkins / Miss E. Gray
1909–38	Miss E. M. Walker
1939–60	Miss G. N. Burbidge
1961–77	Miss V. Bullwinkel

Directors of Nursing

1978–84	Miss M. K. Lafferty
1984–92	Miss V. J. Seeger
1992–96	Miss P. Higginbottom

APPENDIX 3
Nursing Awards, 1963–1989

Year	Dr Doris Officer / Vivian Bullwinkel Prize	Dr McLorinan Prize	Comm. of Management / Board of Management Prize	Sister Ruth Rowan Prize	(Tutor's / Principal Nurse Teacher / Principal Nurse Educator / Nurse Teacher)	Matron's / Nursing Director's / Director of Nursing's Prize
1963/64			L. Taualii; M. Sheen	H. Welter; R. Schraguer		A. Risch
1964/65			M. Anderson	O. Kanitsakis; L. Magin		J. Donehue
1965/66			D. Walshe	S. Blanchard		C. M. Black; B. Marten
1966/67	G. Backman	C. Black; M. Dear	L. Hastwell	P. Seaton		L. Franklin
1967/68	B. Hastwell; S. O'Connor	S. Blanchard; C. Cole	C. Backman	F. Minion; A. Cossio		H. Mitchell; A. Commadeur
1968/69	B. Needham	H. Black; M. Black	A. DEDeugd	J. More	M. Larkins	P. Ryan
1969/70	M. Shaw	A. Commader	G. Iversen	C. Scrimgeour; M. Van Der Klugt	E. Kenny; B. McMillan	D. Urquhart
1970/71	M. Shaw	J. More; D. McAlpine	G. Iversen	C. Scrimgeour; M. Van Der Klugt	E. Evans	D. Urquhart
1971/72	B. Cattapan; S. Withers	R. Jakaitis; J. Maguire	V. Thompson; J. Piajek	L. Dodd	no prize	W. Eadie
1972/73	E. Birkett; N. Tagg	K. Lockwood	C. Humphries	H. Rees	K. Haines	J. Mastwyk
1973/74	?	?	?	?	?	?
1974/75	C. Kelly	J. Mastwyk; N. Tagg	M. Van Der Valk	A. Whitting	E. Dempsey	K. Nessel; P. Milne
1975/76	E. Mayes	K. Burchett; M. Mitchell	A. Leviston; R. Cameron	I. Mayer	K. Ryan	G. Hatherall
1976/77	M. Lee; M. McGough	J. Willis	C. Arnold	C. Finearty	H. Naus	H. Farquhar; J. Hollis
1977/78	J. Brake	H. Johnson	P. Damen	J. Taylor	B. Grant	J. Backland; L. Jordan

1978/79	G. Reid; A. Bennets	E. McGlashen	J. Edmonds	P. Malone	J. Gunn	J. Goudge; D. Skinner
1979/80	G. Phillips	N. Amey	A. Sarget	no prize	H. Esplan	D. Robbins; C. Martin
1980/81	J. Avery; C. Hamilton	K. Slater	K. Meehan	J. Wilkie	D. Stratton	C. Bradshaw; D. Lawson
1981/82	G. Phillips	N. Amey	A. Sarget	no prize	H. Esplan	D. Robbins; C. Martin
1982/83	H. Simpson	C. Pendock	A. Wright	no prize	L. Wallish	D. McCormick; J. Wilson
1983/84	J. Anderson; T. Popple	A. Sargent	C. Wetmore	no prize	G. Crick	C. Emery
				Post Basic Prize	Post Basic Prize	
1984/85	J. Biddlestone	M. Taylor	D. Morrison	B. Milanes	J. Hore	

Untitled General Awards

1985/86	J. Stephens	L. Niklaus	J. Blom	L. Thompson	C. Kennedy	S. Radcliffe
1986/87	F. Hudghton	P. Cashman	C. Le Sueur	L. Ives	L. Pinn	
1987/88	J. Maxwel	Y. TornBroers	G. Houghton	M. O'Sullivan		
1988/89	D. Kiegaldie	J. Sexton	S. White	C. Anderson		
1989/90	J. Roney	E. Bambery	M. Villani			

Treatment Statistics

Admissions/Discharges 1914–1996

Year	Admissions	Discharges	Deaths	Mortality rate
1914/15	1521	1410	62	4.60
1915/16	3077	2809	141	4.68
1916/17	3443	3304	122	3.53
1917/18	3874	3583	137	3.60
1918/19	4879	4795	248	5.00
1919/20	4297	3965	214	5.05
1920/21	4349	4133	157	3.6
1921/22	3568	3653	85	2.3
1922/23	3677	3521	72	1.93
1923/24	3929	3712	119	3.07
1924/25	3450	3492	120	3.40
1925/26	2878	2864	81	2.78
1926/27	3612	3387	78	2.20
1927/28	4243	4130	110	2.59
1928/29	4399	4324	115	2.60
1929/30	4294	4174	116	2.70
1930/31	4954	4704	93	1.91
1931/32	5947	5797	145	2.44
1932/33	5696	5554	104	1.84
1933/34	5065	5077	101	1.97
1934/35	4522	4505	114	2.49
1935/36	5859	5686	102	1.75
1936/37	4053	4058	66	1.61
1937/38	4055	4057	116	2.86
1938/39	3778	3636	50	1.34
1939/40	6756	6462	55	0.84
1940/41	7435	7168	127	1.73
1941/42	4701	4863	79	1.64
1942/43	5209	4951	151	2.93

Year	Admissions	Discharges	Deaths	Mortality rate
1943/44	5599	5595	68	1.20
1944/45	4686	4803	45	0.95
1945/46	3479	3396	65	1.9
1946/47	2964	2946	36	1.21
1947/48	2810	2830	35	1.23
1948/49	4644	4560	57	1.23
1949/50	3853	3762	46	1.28
1950/51	3641	3619	47	1.28
1951/52	3929	3906	47	1.20
1952/53	4405	4445	46	1.02
1953/54	4024	3959	45	1.05
1954/55	4726	4661	41	90
1955/56	4797	4724	73	1.52
1956/57	4218	4208	61	1.44
1957/58	4689	4596	118	2.52
1958/59	5000	4825	137	2.74
1959/60	4969	4867	119	2.39
1960/61	5463	5308	144	2.63
1961/62	6031	5913	127	2.10
1962/63	6181	5961	144	2.32
1963/64	6956	6838	143	2.05
1964/65	6880	6791	135	1.96
1965/66	6355	6238	99	1.55
1966/67	6052	5974	101	1.66
1967/68	6021	5928	99	1.64
1968/69	6341	6218	97	1.52
1969/70	6330	6252	105	1.65
1970/71	5841	5770	103	1.76
1971/72	5788	5713	65	1.12
1972/73	5752	5731	76	1.32
1973/74	5642	5518	87	1.54
1974/75	5921	5851	94	1.58
1975/76	4818	4735	71	1.47
1976/77	4549	4540	62	1.36
1977/78	3961	3907	52	1.31
1978/79	4461	4442	34	0.76
1979/80	3845	3812	28	0.72
1980/81	3463	3427	45	1.29
1981/82	3441	3377	41	1.19
1982/83	3436	3365	82	2.38
1983/84	3053	3023	53	1.73
1984/85	2874	2802	64	2.22

Year	Admissions	Discharges	Deaths	Mortality rate
1985/86	5913★	5863★	62	1.04
1986/87	6687	6642	46	0.68
1987/88	7463	7397	63	0.84
1988/89	9216		89	0.96
1989/90	10,206		89	0.87
1990/91	11,080		114	1.02
1991/92	10,606			
1992/93	10,865			
1993/94	11,114			
1994/95	12,285			
1995/96				

★ From 1985/86, figures include renal dialysis same-day patients but exclude admissions from leave.

Major diseases 1914–1936

Year	Scarlet fever (Scarlatina)	Diphtheria	Measles (Morbilli)	Tuberculosis	Tonsilitis and Pharyngitis	Pneumonia and Bronch- Pneumonia	Whopping cough (Pertusis)	Laryngitis
1914/15								
Admitted	120	1243	83	1	59	1	–	7
Discharged	110	1140	93	–	54	1	–	7
Died	2 (1.72)	63(5.15)		1 (100.)	1 (1.75)	–	–	–
1915/16								
Admitted	394	2478	41	–	102	5	29	8
Discharged	331	2290	39	–	104	2	20	8
Died	8 (2.18)	117 (4.79)	1 (2.47)	–	3 (2.87)	3 (60.)	6 (21.82)	–
1916/17								
Admitted	668	2442	76	–	140	5	39	9
Discharged	608	2377	75	–	138	4	29	9
Died	12 (1.86)	96 (3.90)	3 (3.89)	–	2 (1.43)	1 (20.)	8 (21.05)	–
1917/18								
Admitted	995	2361	83	2	224	10	39	9
Discharged	956	2179	78	–	211	8	29	9
Died	19 (1.91)	59 (2.56)	5 (6.03)	2 (100.)	4 (1,52)	2 (20.)	8 (21.05)	–
1918/19								
Admitted	860	2612	35	–	213	6	34	18
Discharged	934	2649	33	–	217	3	29	15
Died	19 (2.09)	91 (3.41)	1 (2.89)	–	5 (2.30)	3 (50.)	7 (20.)	3 (16.66)

Major diseases 1914–1936 (*cont'd*)

Year	Scarlet fever (Scarlatina)	Diphtheria	Measles (Morbilli)	Tuberculosis	Tonsilitis and Pharyngitis	Pneumonia and Bronch-Pneumonia	Whopping cough (Pertusis)	Laryngitis
1919/20								
Admitted	–	–	289	–	–	–	–	–
Discharge	–	–	340	–	–	–	–	–
Died	–	–	18 (5.56)	–	–	–	–	–
1920/21								
Admitted	–	–	3	3	–	–	–	–
Discharge	–	–	3	3	–	–	–	–
Died	–	–	–	1 (28.6)	–	–	–	–
1921/22								
Admitted	1	2	34	–	–	–	–	–
Discharge	1	2	31	–	–	–	–	–
Died	–	–	3 (8.9)	–	–	–	–	–
1922/23								
Admitted	–	1	113	3	237	–	–	–
Discharge	–	1	76	3	221	–	–	–
Died	–	1 (100.)	5 (5.2)	–	–	–	–	–
1923/24								
Admitted	–	2	70	–	120	–	–	–
Discharge	–	1	94	–	135	–	–	–
Died	–	1 (50.)	4 (4.76)	–	–	–	–	–

1924/25								
Admitted	5	16	40	–	3	–	–	–
Discharge	5	–	43	–	4	–	–	–
Died	–	3 (31.68)	–	–	–	–	–	–
1925/26								
Admitted	7	24	66	–	1	20	–	5
Discharge	6	34	62	–	1	14	–	5
Died	1 (25.)	1 (3.39)	1 (10.91)	–	–	–	–	–
1926/27								
Admitted	4	1	20	–	11	11	1	1
Discharge	3	3	23	–	9	16	1	1
Died	1 (25.)	–	–	–	–	1 (7.1)	–	–
1927/28								
Admitted	2	11	12	–	56	4	1	5
Discharge	2	7	13	–	58	2	1	5
Died	–	–	–	–	–	1 (28.57)	–	–
1928/29								
Admitted	4	19	58	16	17	8	–	9
Discharge	4	18	56	12	16	8	–	8
Died	–	–	1 (1.75)	4 (25.)	–	1 (11.6)	–	1 (11.11)
1929/30								
Admitted	7	–	27	–	4	10	–	1
Discharge	7	3	28	–	5	8	–	1
Died	–	–	–	–	–	2 (20.)	–	–

Major diseases 1914–1936 (*cont'd*)

Year	Scarlet fever (Scarlatina)	Diphtheria	Measles (Morbilli)	Tuberculosis	Tonsilitis and Pharyngitis	Pneumonia and Bronch-Pneumonia	Whopping cough (Pertusis)	Laryngitis
1930/31								
Admitted	9	3	21	3	–	11	–	11
Discharge	9	4	20	2	–	11	–	9
Died	–	–	1 (4.76)	1 (33.33)	–	–	–	–
1931/32								
Admitted	24	–	27	1	–	5	–	6
Discharge	24	1	27	–	–	5	–	8
Died	–	–	–	1 (100.)	–	–	–	–
1932/33								
Admitted	5	–	7	–	–	–	–	–
Discharge	5	–	6	–	–	–	–	–
Died	–	–	–	–	–	–	–	–
1933/34								
Admitted	12	–	22	2	–	14	–	5
Discharge	11	–	23	2	–	15	–	5
Died	–	–	–	–	–	–	–	–

1934/35							
Admitted	18	–	111	–	30	–	6
Discharge	19	–	93	–	27	–	6
Died	–	–	2 (1.94)	–	1 (3.45)	–	–
1935/36							
Admitted	21	–	49	–	26	–	16
Discharge	21	–	61	–	28	–	16
Died	–	–	2 (3.57)	–	–	–	–

APPENDIX 5
Aims and Objectives

From the Annual Report, 1994, p. 2.

1. To be a hospital to afford relief including maintenance, rehabilitation and treatment, care of or attention to any disease or ailment or any injury, medical or surgical attendance, medicine, nursing assistance support or aid of any kind or in any form to persons suffering or suspected of suffering from infectious disease or the residual effects of infectious disease and such other persons as in the opinion of the Board of Management of the hospital are appropriate persons to be patients of the hospital.

2. To provide:
    a. For the teaching, instruction or training of persons including nurses, undergraduate and post-graduate students and medical practitioners, technicians and allied health staff on matters relating to infectious disease or the functions of the hospital.
    b. Educational, advisory and consulting services to the public, industry, commerce, health care institutions, hospitals, government both local and State on matters relating to infectious disease.

3. To provide facilities for and carry out and promote research with respect to infectious diseases in both humans and animals, or the functions of the hospital, by all means and set up equipment and maintain laboratories, offices or other buildings or apparatus for that purpose.

4. To promote and further knowledge in the field of medicine and surgery, especially in relation to infectious disease and, without limiting the generality of the foregoing, to seek to discover the nature, origins, and causes of infectious disease by applying any or all those branches of science which are relevant to this purpose and make use of this knowledge so gained for the improvement of diagnosis, treatment or prevention of infectious disease in both human beings and animals.

5. To apply for, obtain and hold industrial property rights (including, without limiting the generality of the foregoing, patents, copyrights, trademarks and registered designs) arising from relating to or concerning any inventions or discoveries made by or on behalf of the hospital.

6. To commercially exploit any research or intellectual property rights undertaken by or belonging to the hospital and any educational advisory or consulting services provided by the hospital.

7. To disseminate when and if the Board of Management thinks advisable, by printed publication or otherwise, any information or advice concerning any matters relating to infectious disease or the functions of the hospital.

APPENDIX 6
Organisational Structure 1995/96

Board of Management

Finance and Staff Committee
HIV Care Liaison Committee
House Committee
Joint Consultative Committee
Medical Advisory Committee
Patient Review Care Committee
Research and Ethics Committee
Senior Medical Appointments Committee
Special Purposes Medical Fund Committee

Executive Director

Director of Medical Services	Director of Nursing	Internal Auditor	Director of Administrative Services	Director of Financial Services	Director of Marketing
Clinical Services	Chaplaincy Services		Administrative Services	Financial Accounting	Clinical Services Consultant
Dietetics	Graduate Centre for Contemporary Nursing Practice		Centre for Social Health	Management Accounting	Fundraising
Education and Research			Communications	Centre for Health Information Technology	Marketing
Medical Administration	Nursing Services—Clinical		Engineering		Office of International Health
Medical Records	Vivian Bullwinkel Education Centre		Environmental Services, Domestic Linen and Residential	Faircom	Public Relations
Occupational Therapy					Volunteer Auxilliary
Pharmacy			Food Services		
Physiotherapy			Personnel and Payrool		
Radiology			Safety		
Social Work			Security		
Victorian Infectious Diseases Reference Laboratory			Supply		

APPENDIX 7

Fairfield's Legacy, the Victorian Infectious Diseases Reference Laboratory

The Victorian Infectious Diseases Reference Laboratory (VIDRL) is a key Victorian public health reference laboratory. Considerable expertise in the laboratory sciences of infectious diseases and public health are concentrated in the VIDRL complex, together with specialist facilities and valuable reference collections of clinical material, reagents and epidemiological records. The VIDRL is structured into four service areas: Virology, Microbiology and Laboratory Services, Epidemiology and Public Health, and Research and Molecular Development. These inter-related areas combine to provide laboratory-based surveillance of infectious disease, the investigation of outbreaks, specialist testing and advice, as well as developmental research and education programs.

VIDRL is derived from the laboratories of the former Fairfield Hospital, which developed a strong reputation as a centre for excellence in the laboratory science of infectious diseases. VIDRL was formally designated as a public health reference laboratory in 1992. Following the closure of Fairfield Hospital in June 1996, stewardship of VIDRL was won by North Western Health Care Network through a tender process and arising from an initiative by the Public Health Division in the Department of Human Services of the Victorian Government. VIDRL was relocated to a new refurbished facility in North Melbourne in May 1998.

VIDRL is a separate business unit of the North Western Health Care Network and is subject to the policies of that organisation as published from time to time. It is guided by an advisory committee with representation that includes the Department of Human Services and both the public and private pathology sectors. A full Category 1 pathology service is offered, although there is a strong emphasis on medical microbiology, with laboratory areas specifically set aside for processing microorganisms in physical containment (PC) conditions at the PC2, PC3 and PC4 level. The National High Security Quarantine Laboratory is a PC4 level containment facility and is designated by the Commonwealth Government as the laboratory responsible for the specific diagnosis of viral haemorrhagic fevers.

A number of special facilities are required for the complex laboratory work at VIDRL. These include: Polymerase Chain Reaction Suites—a complex of four work areas, each with dedicated equipment, consumables and reagents and capable of a high degree of physical containment from each other; Electron Microscopy Facilities —a specially engineered electron microscopy suite and state of the art Phillips CM12 transmission/scanning electron microscope; two Physical Containment level 3 (PC3) laboratories—the Victorian Mycobacterium Reference Laboratory and the HIV culture facility of the Viral Identification Laboratory (part of State HIV Reference Laboratory) and a Physical Containment level 4 (PC4) laboratory, The National High Security Quarantine Laboratory (NHSQL).

The executive management group consists of the General Manager, the four divisional heads, the Laboratory Operations Manager, the Business Manager and two staff representatives. The executive meets weekly and is chaired by the General Manager. The business of the executive is recorded in the minutes of the meetings, the records of which are held in the office of General Manager. The objectives of VIDRL are to provide, in association with the Victorian Department of Human Services, for the State of Victoria a comprehensive public health laboratory service with an emphasis on laboratory services in specialist diagnosis and reference work, infectious disease outbreak investigation, surveillance, development and evaluation of new technology, research, establishment and maintenance of reference collections, education training and consultation and quality control and quality assurance

The vision of VIDRL is to provide high quality laboratory based infectious diseases services to assist the Department of Human Services and other health care organisations in policy development, implementation and assessment for infectious diseases that threaten the health of Victorians. The VIDRL has an internationally recognised role, being a WHO Collaborating Centre for Virus Reference and Research. Amongst the VIDRL complex is a designated WHO Influenza Laboratory and as part of the WHO global poliomyelitis eradication initiative, VIDRL serves as Australia's National Poliovirus Reference Laboratory for the Western Pacific Region. In addition, the VIDRL provides both training and consultation in biosafety, which is formally recognised in WHO Collaborating Centre status in Biosafety. The laboratories have a number of designated State Reference roles, including the Victorian Mycobacterium Reference Laboratory, the Victorian HIV Reference Laboratory and the Victorian Viral Hepatitis Reference Laboratory. The VIDRL also serves as Australia's National High Security Quarantine Laboratory.

The Division of Virology, VIDRL came into being in June 1997 as part of the reorganisation of VIDRL that followed the successful tender by the then Western Health Network. The division comprises three sections of the former Virology department, VIDRL, the Viral Identification Laboratory, under Dr Chris Birch, Senior Scientist, the Infectious Diseases Serology Laboratory, under Dr Alan Breschkin, Senior Scientist and the Electron Microscopy Laboratory under Dr John Marshall. Dr Michael Catton, former deputy director of VIDRL, was appointed head of this new virology division.

During the first year of the Division's operation the major challenges revolved around the planning of the refurbishment of Jane Bell House in Wreckyn Street, North Melbourne, for the new VIDRL laboratory, and the subsequent move to the new site. Despite the short time lines and the complexities involved, which included designing a new Physical Containment Level 4 facility for the National High Security Quarantine Laboratory, the move took place on schedule on the weekend of 29/30 April 1998. The last specimens were processed at the Fairfield site on Friday, 28 April and work commenced in North Melbourne on Monday, 1 May. Late 1997 was also notable for the renewal of the Virology Division's NATA accreditation. Preparation for the laboratory inspection was coordinated by A/Prof Stephen Locarnini, the NATA Signatory, whose molecular virology laboratory was also involved in the accreditation process. The Virology laboratories successfully passed their last NATA inspection on the Fairfield site in August 1997.

A VIDRL wide strategic planning process was commenced in late 1997/early 1998, and the resulting draft strategic plan articulated a shift in focus for the organisation with primary emphasis on public health orientated programs. Major areas of emphasis for the division of virology were identified as vaccine preventable diseases, especially laboratory support of measles control; respiratory pathogens, especially influenza, blood borne and sexually transmitted diseases, especially HIV; gastroenteritis and food-borne pathogens, especially Norwalk and Norwalk-like viruses; exotic and vector borne diseases, especially viral haemorrhagic fevers and arboviruses; and provision of virology reference laboratory services. A more coherent approach to quality assurance, staff training and development, and provision of statewide services were also signalled in the division of virology's and VIDRL's plans.

Three way collaborations between the Divisions of Virology and Epidemiology and Public Health of VIDRL and the infectious diseases unit of the Department of Human Services to implement community based clinical and laboratory influenza surveillance, and active surveillance of measles have been notable examples of success in the division's public health program approach.

Several joint investigations of blood borne virus transmission together with the molecular Research & Development Division, and DHS have also been among the highlights of the 1998 year for the virology division.

As a consequence of the VIDRL move to North Melbourne the Virology Division's freshly acquired NATA accreditation will require renewal, with a new inspection date scheduled for April 1999. VIDRL has taken the opportunity to seek NATA accreditation as one laboratory for the first time, and to be accredited to the new ISO guide 25 which will become mandatory in the year 2000. This entails a significant reorganisation of VIDRL's operating systems and documentation and consequently a substantial commitment of time and effort VIDRL wide. At the time of writing this remains a major focus of activity for the division of Virology.

With the closure at Fairfield Infectious Diseases Hospital clinical service, throughput decreased markedly. This particularly affected the non-bacteriology services which it was felt needed maintaining to ensure trained staff for the PC4 specimens. The VIDRL's services has been made available to targeted (e.g. STD Travel) clinics. The experience within MALS (including bacteriology, parasitology, immunohaematology and biochemistry) has ensured a comprehensive service is available. Provision of these services also ensures a flow of primary specimens for pursuing public health objectives. As VIDRL, within NWHCN, continues to evolve and focus on strengths, reference activities within MALS such as the MRL and Malaria reference activities continue.

The Epidemiology and Public Health Division was established in 1997 as part of the restructure of VIDRL. Included in the Division from the previous VIDRL structure were the National Polio Reference Laboratory (also one of the three WHO regional reference laboratories for the Western Pacific Region), the World Health Organisation Collaborating Centre for Biosafety and the Information Technology section of VIDRL. Since its establishment the Division has added one staff member to the polio laboratory and a new member of staff has been recruited to work on the evaluation of the nation-wide measles catch-up campaign.

In its first eighteen months, in addition to a range of projects on measles and influenza conducted in close association with the Virology Division, the Epidemiology Division has been conducting a local study of the epidemiology of human parvovirus, a retrospective case study of hepatitis C which may have been acquired by medical procedures, an ongoing study of infectious diseases in long term Laotian settlers and improved surveillance of diseases which result in acute flaccid paralysis, a clinical marker of the circulation of wild poliovirus.

Collaborations have been established with the Victorian Blood Bank, the Women's and Children's Health Care Network, the University of Melbourne and the Victorian Infectious Diseases Services. The Division has strengthened the laboratory's ties with the World Health Organisation through its collaborations on polio eradication, biosafety and, more recently, enhanced measles control.

A number of surveillance initiatives have been established by of the Epidemiology Division. The fortnightly surveillance bulletin from VIDRL which formerly included two weekly surveillance of viral diagnoses at VIDRL has been expanded to include viral, bacterial and parasitic diseases. The bulletin is now posted on the VIDRL homepage, as well as the homepage of the Victorian Division of General Practice from where it can be down-loaded.

The *VIDRL Quarterly* was re-introduced and published for four issues before being merged with the newly established *Victorian Infectious Diseases Bulletin*. The Director of the Epidemiology Division is one of the two founding editors of the new state-wide infectious diseases bulletin, whose editorial group now includes representation from the Macfarlane Burnet Centre and the Microbiological Diagnostic Unit.

The Division maintains the VIDRL homepage, has developed and maintains a polio homepage and co-ordinates CyberMIDG, an electronic mail network that links members of MIDG, the Melbourne Infectious Disease Group. In addition to this, the IT section of the Division is working on the electronic transfer of notifiable disease data, using the internationally accepted HL7 (health level 7) standard. The Epidemiology Division is also developing a collaborative project on the surveillance of nosocomial diseases in Intensive Care Units.

In its first eighteen months the Division received competitive funding for projects on measles, human parvovirus and hepatitis C from the Public Health Division of the Department of Human Services and, in conjunction with the Virology Division, a grant from Roche Pharmaceuticals for influenza surveillance. The Division was also involved in the co-supervision of two public health trainees, two Master of Public Health students and one student who successfully completed a first class honours degree in Medical Science at Monash University. Members of the Division have presented results of their work at national and international meetings and a number of publications have been submitted or are in press.

In the next two years the Epidemiology Division plans to consolidate its links within VIDRL and its external links, to continue to foster a productive working relationship with the Department of Human Services, to build on areas of particular interest, including measles, influenza, nosocomial infections and electronic management of infectious diseases data, and to expand its areas of interest into other aspects of the epidemiology of infectious diseases. New diagnostic laboratory testing technology is evaluated for use and new assays are developed and implemented. Subsequently experience accumulated with new assays in the reference laboratory is shared with other public and private laboratories either directly, or via conference presentations or in the published literature.

A small but productive research group is active in the development of anti-infective agents and the application of new technology to diagnosis and therapeutic monitoring in infectious diseases. Personnel are predominantly postgraduate students from Melbourne, Monash and La Trobe universities with scholarship support. Research financial support is from external funding bodies and through collaborative commercial projects. A research focus provides the diagnostic and reference divisions of VIDRL with valuable access to special expertise and equipment as well as fostering a climate of excellence within the institution.

Clearly VIDRL, very much the direct research descendant of Fairfield, has continued the excellent research and development work undertaken at the hospital over many years and it is particularly pleasant for friends of Fairfield that VIDRL contains a good number of Fairfield-trained and/or ex-Fairfield staff. Through VIDRL, the Fairfield tradition of service and research excellence continues.

Notes

Introduction

[1] J. Cahill, *How the Irish Saved Civilization: The Untold Story of Ireland's Heroic Role, from the Fall of Rome to the Rise of Medieval Europe*, Hodder and Stoughton, London, 1995, p. 172.
[2] Cannon, *Melbourne After the Gold Rush*, pp. 402–8.
[3] J. M. and M. J. Cohen (eds), *The Penguin Dictionary of Quotations*, Penguin, Harmondsworth, 1975, p. 273. For a detailed account of the Black Death see Ziegler, *The Black Death*.
[4] Christie, *Infectious Diseases*, p. 1.
[5] Coe, *Sociology of Medicine*, p. 149.
[6] Pearn and Cobcroft, *Fevers and Frontiers*, p. 152.
[7] Ibid., pp. 149–55.
[8] Ibid., p. 155.
[9] Cannon, *Life in the Cities*, vol. 3, *Australia in the Victorian Age*, pp. 219–20.

1 Fever Hospital 1890–1918

[1] Goldsmid, *The Deadly Legacy*, pp. ix–x.
[2] Ibid., p. xvii.
[3] Haggar, *Australian Colonial Medicine*, p. 97.
[4] See Anderson, *Roads*, p. 10.
[5] *Sydney Morning Herald*, November 1852.
[6] Haggar, *Australian Colonial Medicine*, p. 98.
[7] Ibid., p. 98.
[8] Barrett, *The Inner Suburbs*, p. 55.
[9] Ibid., p. 55.
[10] Hagger, *Australian Colonial Medicine*, p. 101.
[11] Central Board of Health (Victoria), fifteenth Annual Report, 1874, p. 16.
[12] Ibid.
[13] Sandland, The Changing Pattern of Infectious Diseases, p. ?
[14] Graeme Butler and Associates, National Trust of Australia (Victoria), Draft Classification Report: Fairfield Hospital, unpublished, 1996, p. 6.
[15] Ibid.
[16] *Weekly Times*, 15 October 1904, p. 13.
[17] Committee of Management Minutes, Furnishing Sub-committee Minutes, and *Queen's Memorial Infectious Diseases Hospital, Rules Relating To Patients, Adopted 22 September 1904*, all in the Fairfield Hospital Archives.

[18] Graeme Butler and Associates, National Trust of Australia (Victoria), Draft Classification Report: Fairfield Hospital, unpublished, 1996, p. 1.

[19] Ibid., p. 5.

[20] Ibid., p. 6.

[21] See letters to *Argus*, 14 September 1910, p. 12, and 13 August 1912.

[22] Finance Committee Minute Book, 20 October 1913.

[23] Queen's Memorial Hospital, *Annual Report*, 1915.

2 Queen's Memorial Hospital 1919–1947

[1] *Health Bulletin*, no. 112, July–December 1954, p. 19.

[2] Sandland, The Changing Pattern of Infectious Disease, p. 6.

[3] Ibid., p. 7.

[4] *Health Bulletin*, no. 112, July–December 1954, p. 19.

[5] *Fairfield Hospital Victoria, 1904–1954*, p. 3.

[6] Sandland, The Changing Pattern of Infectious Diseases, p. 9.

[7] Ibid., p. 4.

[8] Burchill, *Australian Nurses Since Nightingale*, p. 22.

[9] Macquarie Library, *Encyclopedia of Ideas: Inventions/Concepts/Discoveries From the Wheel to Nuclear Energy*, p. 511.

[10] *Fairfield Hospital Victoria, 1904–1954*, p. 6.

3 Fairfield Hospital 1948–1969

[1] *Fairfield Hospital 1904–1954*, p. 6.

[2] Ibid., p. 7.

[3] Macfarlane Burnet Centre For Medical Research Limited, *Annual Report*, 1991, p. 1.

[4] *Fairfield hospital 1904–1954*, p. 7.

[5] Ibid.

[6] Sandland, The Changing Pattern of Infectious Disease, p. 11.

[7] *Fairfield hospital 1904–1915*, p. 7.

[8] Sandland, The Changing Pattern of Infectious Disease, p. 7.

[9] Ibid., p. 12.

4 Progress and Challenge 1948–1985

[1] *Report of the Committee of Inquiry into Hospital and Health Services in Victoria*, 1976.

[2] Ibid.

[3] Sandland, The Changing Pattern of Infectious Disease, p. 10.

[4] *Age*, 18 November 1978.

[5] *Age*, 31 December 1980.

5 The Fatal Decade 1986–1996

[1] See also Carol Fox, *Industrial Relations in Nursing (Victoria) 1982–1985*, University of New South Wales Press, Sydney, 1989; Burchill, *Australian Nurses Since Nightingale 1860–1990*, pp. 205–12.

[2] MBCMR, *Annual Report*, 1991, p. 1.

3   *Age*, 20 September, 3 October 1990.

4   *Age*, 26 March 1991.

5   *Age*, 7 June 1991.

6   Ibid.

7   *Age*, 2 December 1991.

8   *Age*, 23 July 1992.

9   *Age*, 27 April 1995.

10   Rosemary Kelly Specialist Research Services, *Impact Assessment of the Phase 1 Report of the Metropolitan Hospitals Planning Board: Developing Melbourne's Hospital Network*, prepared for the Health Services Union of Australia, Victoria No. 1 Branch, July 1995, p. 25.

11   A. Murray Sandland, 'Farewell Speech', Sunday 12 May 1996, Fairfield Hospital (copy courtesy of Dr Sandland).

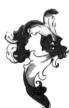

Bibliography

Archival Sources

The Annual Reports of Fairfield Hospital (previously Queen's Memorial Infectious Diseases Hospital) and of the Macfarlane Burnet Centre for Medical Research, together with photographs and miscellaneous material, are held in the Fairfield Hospital Archive athe Austin Hospital, Melbourne.

Secondary Sourcces

Ackernecht, E. H., *History and Geography of the Most Important Diseases*, Hafner, New Your, 1965.

Anderson, W. K., *Roads for the People*, Hyland House, Melbourne, 1994.

Andrew, R. and Barnett, A. (eds), *In Their Day: The Baker Medical Research Institute Memoirs of Alumni*, Hyland House, Melbourne 1992.

Arnold, J. and Morris, D. (eds), *Monash Biographical Dictionary of 20th Century Australia*, Reed, Melbourne, 1994.

Atkinson, J. F., *What Shall We Do With Our Dead?* Melbourne, 1878.

Australian Health Society, *A Twenty-Five Years' Record*, Melbourne, 1900.

Australia Institute of Health, *Australia's Health*, first biennial report of the Australian Institute of Health, Australian Government Publishing Service, Canberra, 1988.

Australian National Council on Aids, Hepatitis C and Related Diseases, hyperlink, http://www.ancahrd.org.au/hiv/index.htm.

Barrett, B., *The Inner Suburbs: The Evolution of an Industrial Area*, Melbourne University Press, Melbourne, 1971.

Barrett, J., *Typhoid Fever in Victoria*, Melbourne, 1883.

Beaumont, J., *Gull Force: Survival and Leadership in Captivity 1941–1945*, Allen & Unwin, Sydney, 1988.

Bickel, L., *The Man Who Made Penicillin*, Sun Papermac, Melbourne, 1983 (first published as *Rise Up to Life*, 1972).

Black, D., *The Plague Years: A Chronicle of AIDS—The Epidemic of our Times*, Picador, London, 1986.

Brogan, A. H., *Committed to Saving Lives: A History of the Commonwealth Serum Laboratories*, Hyland House, Melbourne, 1990.

Burchill, E., *Australian Nurses Since Nightingale 1860–1990*, Spectrum Publications, Melbourne, 1992.

261

Burgmann, V. and Lee, J., *Making a Life: A People's History of Australia since 1788*, McPhee Gribble/Penguin Books, Melbourne, 1988. See in particular 'Keeping the Doctor Away', by John Powles, pp. 70–84.

Burnet, F. M., 'The Natural History of Tuberculosis', *Medical Journal of Australia*, vol. 1, no. 57, 1948.

Campbell, Judy, *Invisible Invaders: Smallpox and other Diseases in Aboriginal Australia, 1780–1880*, Melbourne University Press, Melbourne, 2002.

Cannon, M., *Life in the Cities:*, vol. 3, *Australia in the Victorian Age*, Thomas Nelson, Melbourne, 1975.

Cannon, M., *Melbourne after the Gold Rush*, Loch Haven Books, Main Ridge Vic., 1993.

Carmichael, G. E. J., *Hospital Children: Sketches of Life and Character in the Children's Hospital Melbourne*, Melbourne, 1891.

Cartwright, F. F., *A Social History of Medicine*, Longman, London, 1977.

Charlesworth, M. *et al.* (eds), *Life Among the Scientists: An Anthropological Study of an Australian Scientific Community*, Oxford University Press, Melbourne, 1989.

Christie, A. B., *Infectious diseases: Epidemiology and Clinical Practice*, E & S. Livingstone, Edinburgh, 1969.

Cilento, R., *Tropical Diseases In Australia: A Handbook*, W. R. Smith and Paterson, Brisbane, 1942.

Coates, A. and Rosenthal, N., *The Albert Coates Story: The Will that Found the Way*, Hyland House Melbourne, 1977.

Cochrane, H. C., Penicillin: The Australian Story, unpublished, 1990.

Coe, C. M., *Sociology of Medicine*, McGraw-Hill, Maidenhead UK, 1979.

Cribb, J., *The White Death*, Angus and Robertson, Sydney, 1996.

Cummins, C. (ed.), *Heidelberg Since 1836*, 2nd edn, Heidelberg Historical Society, Melbourne, 1982.

Cumpston, J. H. L., Health and Disease in Australia, edited by Milton Lewis, Australian Government Publishing Service, Canberra, 1989 (completed in 1928 but not published). Cumpston was the first Commonwealth Director General of Health, 1921–1945).

Davis, A. and George, G., *States of Health: Health and Illness in Australia*, 2nd edn, Harper Educational, Sydney, 1993.

Fenner, F., 'Smallpox, "the most dreadful scourge of the human species"', *Medical Journal of Australia*, vol. 141, pp. 728–35, 841–6.

Gibson, G. L., *Infection in Hospital: A Code of Practice*, 2nd edn, Churchill and Livingstone, London, 1974.

Goldsmid, J., *The Deadly Legacy: Australian History and Transmissable Diseases*, New South Wales University Press,/Australian Institute of Biology, Sydney, 1988.

Gould, P., *The Slow Plague: A Geography of the Aids Pandemic*, Blackwell, Cambridge, Mass., 1993.

Hagger, J., *Australian Colonial Medicine*, Rigby, Melbourne, 1979.

Hardy, A., *The Epidemic Streets: Infectious Disease and the Rise of Preventive Medicine, 1856–1900*, Clarendon Press, Oxford, 1993.

Henschen, Folke, *The History of Diseases,* Longmans, London, 1966.

Howe, G. M. (ed.), *A World Geography of Human Diseases*, Academic Press, London, 1977.

Hunter-Payne, G., *Proper Care: Heidelberg Repatriation Hospital 1940s–1990s*, Allen & Unwin, Sydney, 1994.

Karlen, A., *Plague's Progress: A Social History of Man and Disease*, Victor Gollancz, London, 1996 (first published as *Men an Microbes: Disease and Plagues in History and Modern Times*, Putnam Berkley Group, New York, 1995).

Kohn, G. C., *Encyclopedia of Plague and Pestilence*, Wordsworth Reference, New York, 1998.

Lampton, C., *Predicting Aids and Other Epidemics*, Franklin Watts, New York, 1989.

Linge, G. and Porter, D., *No Place for Borders: The HIV/AIDs Epidemic and Development in Asia and the Pacific*, Allen & Unwin, Sydney, 1997.

Mackenna, J. W., *Mortality of Children in Victoria*, Melbourne, 1858.

McCarthy, C., *On the Excessive Mortality of Infants*, Melbourne, 1859.

Mackenna, J. W., *Causes of Diseases of Children*, Melbourne, 1859.

McNeill, W. H., *Plagues and Peoples*, Anchor Press/Doubleday, New York, 1976.

Melbourne General Cemetery: Centenary Souvenir, Melbourne, 1952.

Miller, J., *The Body in Question*, Random House, New York, 1978.

Morris, R. J., *Cholera 1832: The Social Response to an Epidemic*, Holmes and Meier, New York, 1976.

Neild, J. E., *Dirt and Disease*, Melbourne, 1872.

Neild, J. E., *On the Advantages of Burning the Dead*, Melbourne, 1873.

Nikiforuk, A., *The Fourth Horseman: A Short History of Epidemics, Plagues and Other Scourges*, Phoenix, London, 1993.

Pearn, J. and Cobcroft, M., *Fevers and Frontiers*, Amphion Press, Brisbane, 1990.

Petersen, A. and Lupton, D., *The New Public Health: Health and Self in the Age of Risk*, Allen & Unwin, Sydney, 1996.

Pirie, C., *Partnerships in Practice: National HIV/AIDS Strategy, 1996/97 to 1998/99*, Looking Glass Press, **[place??]**, 1996.

Porter, R., *The Greatest Benefit to Mankind: A Medical History of Humanity from Antiquity to the Present*, Fontana Press, London, 1999.

Porter, R. M. and Boag, T. C., *The Australian Tuberculosis Campaign: 1948–1976*, Menzies Foundation, n.d., n.p., *c.* 1990–91.

Price, A. G., *Importance of Disease in History*, Libraries Board of South Australia, Adelaide, 1964.

Proust, A. J., *History of Tuberculosis in Australia, New Zealand and Papua New Guinea*, Brolga Press, Canberra, 1991.

Rich, A. R., *Pathogenesis of Tuberculosis*, C. Thomas, Chicago, 1944.

Rosebury, T., *Microbes and Morals: A Study of Venereal Disease*, Paladin, St Albans UK **[??]**, 1975.

Sandland, A. M., The Changing Pattern of Infectious Diseases, unpublished.

Secretary of State for the Colonies, *Report on Leprosy by the Royal College of Physicians*, HMSO, London, 1867.

Sexton, C., *Burnet: A Life*, Oxford University Press, Melbourne, 1999.

Smith, K. M., *Viruses*, Cambridge University Press, Cambridge, 1962.

Spencer, M., *Malaria: The Australian Experience 1843–1991*, Australasian College of Tropical Medicine, James Cook University of North Queensland, Townsville, 1994.

Sprott, G., *Cause and Prevention of Typhoid Fever*, Hobart, 1898.

Stamp, L. D., *The Geography of Life and Death*, Collins / Fontana Library, London, 1964.

Starobinski, J. A., *History of Medicine*, 2nd edn, Leisure Arts, London, 1965.

Timewell, E., Minichiello, V. and Plummer, D., *AIDS in Australia*, Prentice Hall, Sydney, 1992.

Victoria, Department of Health and Community Services, *Eliminating Tuberculosis: A Strategy for Victoria*, Health and Community Services, Melbourne, *c.* 1996.

Welch, J. H., *Hell to Health: The History of Quarantine at Port Phillip Heads 1852–1966*, The Peninsula Story, Book 2, Nepean Historical Society, Sorrento, 1969.

Wills, C., *Plagues: Their Origin History and Future*, Flamingo, London, 1996.

World Health Organisation, June 2000 hyperlink, http://www.who.int.

Ziegler, P., *The Black Death*, Pelican, Harmondsworth, 1970.

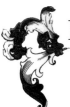

Index

Italic type indicates illustrations. **Bold** type indicates substantial biographies and disease descriptions.

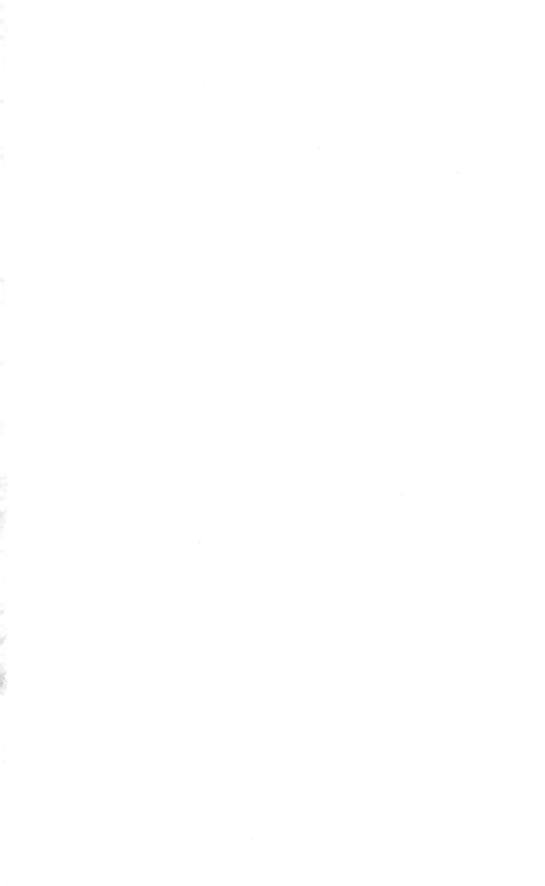